The Identification, Assessment, and Treatment of Adults Who Abuse Animals

T0276053

Kenneth Shapiro • Antonia J.Z. Henderson

The Identification, Assessment, and Treatment of Adults Who Abuse Animals

The AniCare Approach

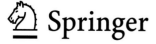 Springer

Kenneth Shapiro
Animals and Society Institute
Washington Grove
MD, USA

Antonia J.Z. Henderson
Department of Psychology
Langara College
Vancouver
BC, Canada

Previous editions originally been published by the society under the title: "The AniCare Model of Treatment for Animal Abuse" (1998).

ISBN 978-3-319-27360-0   ISBN 978-3-319-27362-4   (eBook)
DOI 10.1007/978-3-319-27362-4

Library of Congress Control Number: 2016932523

Springer Cham Heidelberg New York Dordrecht London

Springer International Publishing AG Switzerland is part of Springer Science+Business Media (www.springer.com)

The Identification, Assessment, and Treatment of Adults Who Abuse Animals

The AniCare Approach

by
Kenneth Shapiro, PhD, ABPP
and
Antonia J.Z. Henderson, PhD

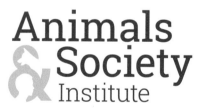

A Project of the Animals and Society Institute
2nd Edition, 2015; 1st Edition, 1998

Acknowledgments

We gratefully acknowledge the Kenneth A. Scott Foundation for the major funding in support of various projects that made the development of this second edition of the handbook possible.

We also are appreciative to the following practitioners who colead or hosted workshops over the years through which we gained insight into the AniCare Adult Approach: Nancy Bell, Cheryl Durbin, Maya Gupta, Lynn Kegley, Wendy McSparren, Mary Lou Randour, Karen Schaefer, Sharon Scott, Karen Stockham, RaeAnn Taylor, Elizabeth Strand, Tamara Ward, and Melissa Winkle.

The following individuals provided editorial suggestions for this edition: Phil Arkow, Anna Chur-Hansen, Catherine Faver, Maya Gupta, Bill Henry, Lori Kogan, Lisa Lunghofer, Mary Lou Randour, Chris Risley-Curtiss, Tania Signal, and Suzanne Tallichet. Cindy Milburn of the International Foundation for Animal Welfare provided input for the material on compassion.

Finally, we are grateful to the many researchers whose studies have provided empirical and theoretical support for the ongoing development of instruments for the identification, assessment, and treatment of adults who abuse animals.

Contents

Introduction

1

1.1 Introduction to the Second Edition

Welcome to the second edition of the adult version of the AniCare Approach to the assessment and treatment of animal abuse.[1] In the first edition of the handbook (Jory and Randour 1998), we framed the "AniCare Approach" through an adaptation of Brian Jory's Intimate Justice theory for perpetrators of domestic violence (Jory and Anderson 1999; Jory et al. 1997). That approach focused on the way clients refuse to accept responsibility for their abuse of animals. Like other violent and antisocial behaviors, there are many pathways to the behavior of animal abuse, as well as many various forms of animal abuse and of animal abuser psychology. Consequently, other subpopulations of animal abusers require other complementary and/or alternative forms of intervention.

Adults who abuse animals are not a monolithic group. The population varies in form and severity of animal abuse (torture, neglect, and killing), presence of psychological issues (degree of pathology and presence of comorbid conditions such as addictions and personality disorders), and role of extra-psychological issues (economically motivated, response to resource depletion, situationally determined responses). Although animal abuse may be the primary presenting problem (e.g., when treatment is court ordered), clients typically present this behavior within a complex context of other individual and systemic (family- and subculturally-based) problems.

For these reasons, AniCare Adult cannot be a cohesive, unitary, one-size-fits-all handbook. Rather, the more modest goal is to provide a set of tools that are useful in and can be adapted for the treatment of the various presentations of this problem behavior.

This greatly expanded second edition is based on empirical literature on the psychology of animal abuse (Ascione and Shapiro 2009), our experience in presenting

---

[1] *AniCare* is derived from the root word *ani,* which means *bring to life* (as in "animate" and, by extension, "animal"), and *care.*

© Springer International Publishing Switzerland 2016

K. Shapiro, A.J.Z. Henderson, *The Identification, Assessment, and Treatment of Adults Who Abuse Animals: The AniCare Approach,*
DOI 10.1007/978-3-319-27362-4_1

over 70 workshops on the AniCare Adult and AniCare Child (Shapiro et al. 2014), and other contemporary innovations in therapy. We begin with a critical review of the literature on the relationships between human violence and animal abuse and an expanded section on the identification and assessment of animal abuse. The remaining sections are organized in the rough sequence of phases of an individual counseling intervention but geared to the presenting problem of animal abuse—framing the therapy, establishing accountability, and teaching empathy, compassion, and other interpersonal skills. We present hoarding, a form of abuse with its own dynamics and demographics, in Sect. 4.4.

In addition to illustrative case material, a number of "exercises" and homeworks are interspersed throughout the text. Although therapists may use their own preferred style, the general posture of the therapist suggested for the exercises is active and directive. The first two exercises come within the initial framing phase of the therapy and are part of the important task of forming a working therapeutic relationship. Later exercises focus on interpersonal skills and are familiar as variations of interventions in a cognitive behaviorist approach—here, adapted for the problem of animal abuse.

Consistent with the variability of the target population, the theoretical basis of the assessment instruments and intervention in this second edition of the handbook, then, is eclectic, replacing Intimate Justice Theory with recent developments in cognitive behaviorism and trauma-based theory as well as aspects of attachment and psychodynamic theories. However, the approach is more case driven and more reliant on nuts-and-bolts responses to the individual client than on theory-based interventions.

In response to the greater recognition among relevant stakeholders of the relationships between violence toward humans and animal abuse and subsequent changes in policy and practice, the handbook now includes materials that address identification, reporting, risk assessment, and diagnostic evaluation in an expanded section on assessment. For this reason, personnel in education, criminal justice, and veterinary medicine also will find the handbook useful.

The handbook, then, can be used by different lay and professional audiences in a number of ways and for a number of purposes: (1) to identify and assess adults who abuse animals, (2) as the primary approach to working with some subpopulations of animal abusers, (3) as a set of tools to be added to a therapist's existing toolbox, and/ or (4) as an intervention that complements a broader treatment program.

We intend this second edition of the handbook to provide a self-guided training, at least for experienced therapists. To this end, we incorporate throughout the text references to a Demonstration DVD (Animals and Society Institute 2001) with role-played interventions, case material (both in the body of the text and in Sect. 4.1), and integration with the recently published second edition of AniCare Child (Shapiro et al. 2014).

To obtain these complementary materials and information about consultations on cases involving AniCare, contact us at:

Animals and Society Institute
2512 Carpenter Road, Suite 202-A
Ann Arbor, MI 48108-1188

By telephone at:
734-677-9240
or e-mail at:
ken.shapiro@animalsandsociety.org

or visit our website at:
www.animalsandsociety.org

1.2 The Violence Connection

Since Tapia's groundbreaking prospective study from 1971 to 1977 (Rigdon and Tapia 1977; Tapia 1971), linking childhood animal abuse with other aggressive behaviors (e.g., destructiveness, fighting, stealing, chaotic home life, and aggressive parenting), a growing and robust literature has demonstrated a convincing association between animal cruelty and other forms of violent behaviors directed at humans. This association, the "violence connection," has emerged in various configurations, coalescing into a comprehensive and persuasive picture.

Since this manual concerns adult-perpetrated animal abuse, the focus of this literature review will examine how the violence connection manifests itself in adult animal cruelty and other antisocial behavior. However, it is worth a brief overview to touch on how the violence connection has been demonstrated in the relationship between animal abuse and deviant behavior in children. Childhood animal abuse may co-occur with other forms of aggression and destructive behavior such as setting fires, bullying, and sexual aggression (Becker et al. 2004; Dadds and Fraser 2006). Children who abuse animals are also more likely to show a lack of empathy, low emotional affect, and callousness—traits that are also linked to psychopathy (Ascione and Shapiro 2009). Animal abuse is also more likely in children who have been abused themselves (Currie 2006) or witnessed intimate partner violence (IPV) between their caregivers (Duncan et al. 2005). Retrospective reports of those convicted of violent criminal acts against humans (assault, rape, and murder) indicate an overrepresentation of childhood acts of animal cruelty. Hensley and Tallichet (2009) found that at least half of their sample of violent offenders reported that they had hit, kicked, or shot animals as children. Regression analyses revealed that drowning and having sex with animals in childhood were predictive of later interpersonal violence as adults. The association between childhood animal cruelty and later deviant behavior is significantly robust such that childhood animal abuse has been included as one criterion for childhood conduct disorder in the Diagnostic and Statistical Manual, Fifth Edition (American Psychiatric Association 2013). Since evidence of conduct disorder with onset before age 15 years is a criterion of adult antisocial personality disorder (ASPD), animal cruelty is also an integral component of this diagnosis. The childhood link and its assessment and treatment are dealt with in more detail in AniCare Child (Shapiro et al. 2014). See also McPhedran (2009) for a review of animal abuse, family violence, and child well-being.

1.2.1 Animal Abuse and Male-Perpetrated Intimate Partner Violence (IPV)

In a groundbreaking study, Ascione (1998) collected self-report data on 38 women living in a battered women's shelter, 28 of whom currently owned pets or had done so within the last year. Fully 71 % of these women reported that their violent partners had also threatened violence toward their pet, and 57 % reported that their partner had actually harmed or killed their animal, including starving, denying veterinary attention, drowning, and setting the animal on fire.

Ascione's findings have been corroborated in subsequent research suggesting that men who perpetrate violence against their partners also perpetrate violence against their pets (or control partners by threatening violence). Rates vary across studies, but at least half and as many as 75 % (Flynn 2011) of women in shelters report that their partner has threatened or committed violence, often egregious violence, against their companion animal. And a sizeable percentage of these women (20–48 % across studies) report that their fear for their animal's safety prolonged their stay in the abusive relationship.

Ascione expanded upon these findings in a larger and more recent (2007) study that focused on pet owners exclusively and included a control group: He found that abused women were 11 times more likely (54 %) than controls (5 %) to report that their partner also abused their family pet. In 72 % of the cases, the harm to the animal was severe involving injury, pain, torture, permanent loss of function, and death. Furthermore, those women whose pets had been abused also experienced more frequent and more extreme violence from their partners than those whose pets had not been abused. In line with previous research, many of the women (18 %) reported that their fear for their pet's safety had prolonged their remaining in the abusive relationship and not seeking refuge at a shelter. Febres et al. (2012) have suggested that an abusive partner's propensity for maladaptive coping in one setting (such as being aggressive toward animals) may be consistent across other settings (such as aggression toward intimate partners).

Other research has also reported on male perpetrators' threatened violence toward family pets as a form of coercion or control. In one study, abusive partners used threats of violence against the victim's pet in order to coerce their partner to commit a crime (Loring and Bolden-Hines 2004). In a 2007 Texas study of 1283 women seeking shelter from domestic violence, Simmons and Lehmann (2007) found that perpetrators who were violent to their partners, and also abused the family pet, utilized a greater range and severity of aggressive violence, including psychological and sexual abuse and stalking. They also reported that the men who abused both their partners and animals engaged in more controlling behavior than men who did not. Upadhya (2014) notes that abusers often exploit the bond that their victims share with their animals and threaten to harm or kill the animal as a means of emotionally abusing their human victim, to establish control, seek revenge, coerce compliance with a demand, or prevent the victim from leaving the relationship. Based on her findings where victims describe their intense anguish at witnessing the torture of their beloved companion animals at the hands of an abusive partner, Upadhya advocates for including this kind of animal abuse as a form of domestic violence. She notes that victims are left increasingly vulnerable to physical and psychological harm through the chronic abuse of their companion animal, may remain in an abusive relationship to protect it, and when they do successfully leave may return for fear of the animal's continued safety. To date, seven states have enacted laws making acts or threats of violence against animals within the definition of domestic violence: Arizona, Colorado, Indiana, Maine, Nebraska, Nevada, and Tennessee.

Victims are often isolated from human social support by their abusive partners. Thus, the animal may fulfill a particularly salient role as an attachment figure, safe haven, and source of emotional support, making the harm or threat of harm to that animal even more poignant. Although the animal bears the scars of the physical abuse, more often the ultimate target of that abuse is the human victim.

> As the victim's social support dwindles, mutual empathy between the human and the animal grows, and feelings of guilt and responsibility for the animal's suffering manifest themselves. The resultant strengthening of the bond between victim and animal may then increase the likelihood and severity of its exploitation. (Upadhya 2014, p. 1177)

1.2.2   Animal Abuse and Female-Perpetrated Intimate Partner Violence (IPV)

The robust finding that women are equally, or slightly more, likely to be perpetrators of IPV than are men has been well supported in the literature since Straus and Gelles first reported this phenomenon in a national survey more than 23 years ago (Straus and Gelles 1988; Archer 2000; Dutton et al. 2005; Magdol et al. 1997; Moffitt et al. 2001). Furthermore, much evidence disconfirms the notion that women's aggression occurs primarily in the context of self-defense against an abusive male partner (Dutton et al. 2005). For example, in a US national survey, Stets and Straus (1989) found that women were three times more likely to use severe violence against a nonviolent male partner (9.6 % in married couples to 13.4 % in cohabiting couples) than were men against a nonviolent female partner (2.3 % in married couples and 1.2 % in cohabiting). This unilateral female-perpetrated IPV argues strongly against a self-defense interpretation. In the past number of years, a large body of research has emerged indicating that women perpetrate violence at similar rates to males and that this trend is consistent across dating, cohabiting, and marital relationships. Research indicates that there are even higher rates of aggression, particularly for women, in young dating couples. In one of the few prospective studies to examine violence in intimate relationships, Magdol et al. (1997) followed a birth cohort of 1037 participants in Dunedin, New Zealand, and found that both minor and severe physical violence rates were higher for women regardless of which member of the couple was reporting. Females' severe violence rates were actually triple that of males (18.6 % vs. 5 %). In a comprehensive meta-analysis, Archer (2000) reports that it is not only low-risk acts that are perpetrated by women, but that a substantial minority of endorsements of "beat up" and "choke or strangle" involved women perpetrators. For decades political correctness and concerns that the reporting of female perpetration of abuse would undermine support for female victims of IPV have been instrumental in silencing these findings and have effectively, albeit unwittingly, stalled progress in addressing this widespread issue; Archer (2000) notes that concern for women victims is not misplaced, as there is also strong evidence for male perpetration of IPV. However, regarding women as the *only* victims of partner violence fails to recognize that anyone who is subjected to chronic and systematic violence is likely to suffer both physical and psychological consequences; this is equally true for men as it is for women. Indeed, men may suffer additional problems associated with a lack of recognition and corresponding support for their situation (Hines et al. 2007).

Interestingly, as discussed later in this handbook (pp. xx), gender plays a different role in the perpetration of violence against animals, with higher rates of animal abuse reported among men, higher rates of animal hoarding reported among women, and approximately equal rates of animal neglect.

The violence connection literature has been slow to talk about women's violence and its relationship to animal cruelty. Indeed, the keyword "female perpetrator" is notably absent from virtually all "violence connection" or "violence link" related journal articles. One notable exception is the work of Febres et al. (2012) study of 87, predominantly Caucasian, women, court referred to batterer intervention programs. As predicted, female perpetrators of IPV, much like male perpetrators, demonstrated much higher rates of animal abuse (17 %) than has been reported in the general population (0.28 %; Vaughn et al. 2009). A variety of physically aggressive acts toward animals were reported along with psychological aggression including threatening, scaring, intimidating, and bullying. Women who reported having committed animal abuse also reported higher rates of perpetrated physical and psychological violence toward their partners than women who reported no animal abuse.

Future research on the violence connection needs to acknowledge that women are equally capable and culpable of perpetrating IPV and animal cruelty, and begin to uncover the complex relationship between perpetrated IPV and animal abuse in women as well as men.

1.2.3 Animal Abuse and Other Forms of Criminality

Retrospective reports of criminal offenders indicate that violent offenders report significantly higher levels of having abused animals (including severe torture and killing) as children than nonviolent offenders (i.e., those involved in drug-related crimes, illegal possession of weapons, or property crimes) (Ascione 2001; Ascione et al. 2007; Kellert and Felthous 1985; Merz-Perez et al. 2001). Much of the research linking animal abuse to other forms of criminality is subsumed under one or the other of two hypothesis or theories to explain the etiology of this link: the graduation hypothesis and the deviance generalization hypothesis.

1.2.3.1 Graduation Hypothesis and Deviance Generalization Hypothesis

The violence graduation hypothesis as used elsewhere in the literature to explain the etiology of antisocial behaviors is sometimes employed in relation to animal abuse. It proposes a direct causal link between early childhood abuse of animals and later adult criminal violence against humans. The hypothesis suggests that childhood animal abuse allows the offender to learn about, practice, and become desensitized to violence directed at a living victim and thus provides a rehearsal ground for later acts of violence directed at humans (e.g., Wright and Hensley 2003). The graduation hypothesis is based upon two central tenets that (1) violence directed at animals precedes that of violence directed at humans and that (2) this graduation from childhood animal cruelty to adult human-directed violence is specific to adult violent offending and not to other nonviolent criminal activity (Ascione 2001; Gullone et al. 2003; Volant et al. 2008; Walters 2013).

Much of the support for the graduation hypothesis comes from research looking at particularly egregious forms of adult violent offending and finding that many of these criminals had childhood histories of severe animal cruelty. For example, Wright and Hensley (2003) looked at five high-profile serial killers and found that 21 % of the 354 serial murders they examined displayed evidence of animal abuse rehearsal in childhood, often using similar methods of killing both their animal and human victims. Wright and Hensley suggest that these criminals had learned to use killing as a way to resolve intolerable psychological states of powerlessness and rage.

Subsequent research has criticized the graduation hypothesis, however. Walters (2013) notes that there are many children who abuse animals who do not go on to become serial murderers, and as Wright and Hensley's research itself illustrates, there are many serial murderers who did not abuse animals as children (in their study only 21 % of the serial murders were correlated with childhood animal cruelty; 79 % were not). Walters' comprehensive meta-analysis of 19 studies found that although there appears to be a link between childhood animal cruelty and later criminal offending, this link is not specific to violent offending (2013). When the data were analyzed as a "within subjects" design rather than the typical "between subjects" design of previous studies, animal cruelty was found to correlate equally well with nonviolent offending as it did with violent offending.

Arluke et al. (1999) proposed the deviance generalization hypothesis as an alternative to the violence graduation hypothesis. According to this view animal cruelty is one component of a larger construct of deviance. A wide range of antisocial behaviors tend to be associated with one another possibly because one behavior leads to another, but more likely because they all stem from common underlying sources. The deviance generalization hypothesis makes no assumptions about a sequential order of deviance (such as violence toward animals leading to human violence and thus necessarily preceding it) and does not assume that animal cruelty leads only to *violent* criminal offending.

Arluke tested this hypothesis analyzing the criminal records of 153 convicted animal abusers and 153 controls who had no history of animal abuse. In support of the deviance generalization hypothesis, he found that animal cruelty was more likely to follow interpersonal violence (56 %) as to precede it (44 %) and just as likely to be associated with nonviolent offending as violent offending.

More recently Febres et al. (2014), in a study of 307 men arrested for IPV, found that 41 % had committed at least one act of animal abuse since the age of 18. This compares to a 1.5 % prevalence rate for men in the general population. These researchers looked not only at a history of animal abuse but also at other variables found to be strongly associated with IPV in previous research, such as traits of antisocial personality disorder (ASPD) and alcohol abuse. Although they found a strong correlation between a history of animal abuse and IPV, animal abuse did not significantly predict IPV perpetration above and beyond ASPD traits and alcohol use. These findings suggest that IPV may be driven by a constellation of factors, one of which is abuse directed at animals. The authors stress that future research is needed in order to disentangle the complicated relationship among various factors associated with both animal abuse and IPV.

Arluke contends that because his and other studies disconfirm the violence graduation hypothesis, this in no way trivializes the very real problem of animal cruelty. Indeed, animal cruelty seems to be linked with a whole range of antisocial behavior including, but not limited to, violence directed at humans. Individuals who commit even one single act of animal cruelty (acts much less heinous and sensationalized than those of the serial murderer subjects in much of the graduation hypothesis literature) are more likely to be involved in other kinds of criminal offending than matched participants who do not abuse animals. These results suggest that even more concern needs to be directed to any degree of animal abuse as a potential red flag of other antisocial behavior and that a more nuanced understanding of this complex relationship is warranted than that offered by the graduation hypothesis.

1.2.4   Animal Abuse and Self-Harm

Vaughn et al. (2015), in a nationally representative community sample of more than 34,000 US residents representing all 50 states, looked at whether people who deliberately harm themselves—"Have you ever cut, scratched, or burned yourself on purpose?"—also harm others. Almost 3 % of respondents ($n = 526$) reported that they had deliberately injured themselves. As predicted, these individuals were also more likely to engage in a variety of violent behaviors including robbery, IPV, forcing sex on another, use of a weapon, and cruelty to animals. The authors suggest that this link between deliberate self-harm and other forms of violent behavior may well be fueled by negative emotionality coupled with poor emotion regulation.

1.2.5   Policy Implications

Indeed, this review is but a small sampling of a very robust literature indicating that violence toward animals and other kinds of antisocial behavior covary. The next questions then are: how have and how should these findings impact policy decisions? Ascione and Shapiro (2009) suggest the paradigm of primary, secondary, and tertiary prevention as a way to review and organize existing and proposed policy about animal abuse and its link to antisocial behavior.

Primary prevention refers to education of the larger community in an effort to deflect problems before they occur. Examples include elementary school training in empathy and compassion that focuses on attitudes toward animals and care and responsibility for animals in the home.

Arbour et al. (2009) in a literature review of Humane Education Programs (HEP) note that despite the existence of over 2000 such programs currently operating in the USA, there is scant research about the efficacy of teaching children about humane animal treatment and empathy-building skills on their subsequent attitudes and behavior toward animals. They examined the efficacy of a specifically designed (HEP) in 37 fourth-grade students in Queensland, Australia. Experimental groups received two 1-h lessons per week for 4 weeks focusing on general animal husbandry and care and animal cruelty. Interestingly, the intervention had more impact on boys than on girls. The authors suggest that boys may be a useful target group for HEP, particularly given that boys are overrepresented in the commission of deliberate animal cruelty.

The advancement of Human-Animal Studies (HAS) as a graduate and postgraduate degree in many universities, most of which include a comprehensive component on the violence connection, is another example of primary prevention. HAS has provided an academic legitimacy to the study of animals, animal abuse, and animal/human relationships and promoted policy development and practices that maximize benefits and minimize costs to both parties. In this way, HAS performs a role much like other movements have done for other oppressed groups, to reveal how animals have been constructed and used throughout history, and offer new ways of interaction to reduce and eventually end chronic discrimination and exploitation.

Secondary prevention focuses on identifying those at risk of committing violent acts toward animals or humans and the implementation of a wide range of preventative and remedial programs aimed at curtailing further animal abuse and/or human-directed violence. Being able to correctly identify "at-risk" populations is key to effective secondary prevention. One such strategy involves networking across agencies, initiating cross-reporting and cross-training protocols to teach human service workers how to recognize and report perpetrators and victims of animal abuse, and, concurrently, teaching animal humane service personnel to recognize child, spousal, and elder abuse (National Link Coalition 2015a).

Identification of at-risk populations at an early age or stage of abuse (before animal abuse has become systemic) allows for more effective intervention. Although the graduation hypothesis (that animal abuse necessarily precedes and leads to later violence enacted upon humans) has not been substantiated in the literature, co-occurrence of animal and human abuse has received strong research support and underlines the need for early identification, regardless of whether human-directed violence has preceded, is co-occurring, or follows the abuse directed at animals.

Mandatory reporting by veterinarians of suspected animal abuse is one such method of identification and a topic of significant debate within the veterinary profession (Babcock and Neihsl 2006; Lofflin 2006) and mental health community. This debate includes concerns about confidentiality and the possibility that mandated reporting might reduce the likelihood of a pet owner seeking care for an injured animal (similar to concerns raised by pediatricians when mandated reporting of suspected child maltreatment was first proposed). Despite these potential drawbacks, mandatory or permissive reporting by veterinarians of animal abuse, with protections from civil and criminal liability, as 20 states have enacted, could enable interventions that may prevent further animal abuse and/or human violence. Two states—California and Colorado—mandate that veterinarians report suspected child abuse, and Illinois does likewise for elder abuse. Eighteen states require everyone to report suspected child abuse, but veterinarians typically have not received training about this requirement.

As discussed earlier, since many victims of IPV do not leave abusive relationships for fear of what will happen to their companion animals, a key policy concern is the development of shelters for animals as well as their human guardians. Ideally, shelters that can also accommodate victim's companion animals offer the best alternative. Victims may be particularly reliant on the comfort and support provided by their companion animals after the trauma of leaving an abusive relationship. Some 100 domestic violence shelters now are pet friendly and allow companion animals to accompany their persons, through the SAFT (Sheltering Animals and Families Together) program. Alternatively, cooperative arrangements between women's shelters, animal shelters, and veterinary facilities, so-called safe havens, provide secure housing for victims' companion animals and thereby decrease the likelihood that victims remain in abusive situations to protect their animals (Carlisle-Frank and Flanagan 2006; Ascione 2000). Domestic violence shelter personnel are also more frequently gathering information about companion animals at intake interviews and considering these animals in safety plans that allow victims to escape imminent abusive situations.

Additionally, programs that identify at-risk youth, and have them work directly with animals in need, show much potential in the realm of effective secondary prevention. For example, Project Second Chance (Harbolt and Ward 2001) pairs at-risk youth with shelter dogs to train the dogs in basic obedience and thereby enhance the dogs' adoptability. In turn the dogs teach the youth about care, attachment, and empathy—skills which are often missing from their problematic histories.

Tertiary prevention involves direct intervention with those who have demonstrated deviant and/or illegal behavior. Recommended or mandated psychotherapy for convicted animal abusers is now included in the anticruelty statues in 34 states. To date seven states have specifically criminalized animal abuse committed with the intention to harm a family member (Upadhya 2014).

This recognition of animal abuse as treatable issue that can benefit from psychological intervention has led to the development of assessment and treatment models such as the one presented in this AniCare manual. Together with the corresponding model for treatment of juveniles (Shapiro et al. 2014), they offer a psychological paradigm and intervention techniques for working with adults and juveniles, presenting with the problem of animal abuse. Notably, individuals presenting with animal abuse vary considerably in their level of psychopathology, and no one treatment approach will be appropriate for all animal abusers.

Identification and Assessment

2

In this chapter, we discuss the identification, assessment, and referral of individuals who have abused or are at risk of abusing animals. Once identified, assessment and referral are necessary. While focusing on human service providers, we also discuss the role of other professions and interest groups, such as criminal justice, veterinary medicine, and education. Where appropriate, assessment can include use of a screening device, general assessment for precursor and comorbid conditions and disorders, and assessment specific to the behavior of animal abuse. We begin with a critical review of definitional issues and descriptions of several schemas on animal abuse and abuser types.

2.1   Defining Abuse

Defining animal abuse should be straightforward. However, several complicating considerations should inform efforts to identify individuals for whom an assessment should be undertaken. Social scientific, legal, and animal advocacy definitions of animal abuse are different, influence each other, and change over time.

> Each individual has his or her own definitions based upon personal experiences, upbringing, cultural standards, spiritual beliefs, and other standards. These definitions are organic and change over time and situational contexts. (Arkow and Lockwood 2013)

A definition from the social scientific literature is as follows: Animal abuse is "...non-accidental, socially unacceptable behavior that causes pain, suffering or distress to and/or the death of an animal" (Ascione and Shapiro 2009, p. 570). This definition replaces the term "intentional" with the term "non-accidental" used by the same first author in an earlier publication (Ascione 1993, p. 228). The more recent term more clearly includes neglect, the most common form of animal abuse. Neglect can involve extreme suffering as, for example, in a case where failure to provide food to two dogs chained in the backyard lead to cannibalization of one dog

© Springer International Publishing Switzerland 2016
K. Shapiro, A.J.Z. Henderson, *The Identification, Assessment, and Treatment of Adults Who Abuse Animals: The AniCare Approach*,
DOI 10.1007/978-3-319-27362-4_2

by the other. More critically for our purposes, neglect resulting in such egregious consequences is often indicative of serious problems in the responsible caretaker.

Also, note that the definition limits "animal abuse" to "socially unacceptable behavior." The findings on the relationship between human violence and animal abuse summarized in the general introduction are based on socially *unacceptable* behaviors by individuals acting primarily in domestic settings, while the treatment of animals in commercial and public institutional settings (agriculture, entertainment, and research) is largely excluded. The recent success of animal protection organizations in challenging some practices in these latter settings narrows the range of socially and legally acceptable treatment of animals. For example, a California statute addresses issues such as crating of veal calves and the use of battery cages for chickens (California and Health and Safety Code Act of 2008).

Still, aside from aberrations in currently acceptable practices by individuals in those institutional settings, the task of identifying individuals who abuse animals and who should be assessed for possible human service intervention is, appropriately, largely confined to those acting in the home and neighborhood. Even in these latter contexts, what is socially unacceptable is continually changing. For example, obesity in animals which reduces activity and increases the likelihood of illness is getting more attention and may come to be recognized as a form of neglect. The Association for Pet Obesity Prevention (2015) reports that between 50 and 60 % of cats and dogs in the United States are overweight or obese.

Finally, Ascione's definition includes and distinguishes suffering and death. Whether nonhuman animals are capable of suffering has been a contentious topic in the contemporary debate over our treatment of them. However, based on findings in cognitive ethology and neuroscience, the attribution of suffering to animals has become accepted in academic writings and public attitudes. Similarly, particularly in moral philosophy, while the ethics of a painless death have been debated, few philosophers argue that an unnecessary death, even if painless, is acceptable. Statements such as—"it is only an animal; animals don't suffer; the animal died without feeling a thing…."—may no longer be socially acceptable in many circles.

As of March 2014, all 50 states in the United States had enacted statutes which make at least some forms of animal abuse a felony. "Animal cruelty," the preferred term for animal abuse in legal contexts, emphasizes the motivation of the perpetrators rather than the harm done to the animal victims. While laws vary from state to state, statutory definitions of animal cruelty typically involve the following language: "Intentionally and maliciously killing, injuring, maiming, torturing, burning, or mutilating" (Kansas and Crimes against the Public Morals 2009). By contrast, crimes only rising to the level of misdemeanors refer to "intentionally abandoning" or "intentionally failing to provide food, water, shelter, exercise, and other care." Note that both intention and malice are required at the level of a felony and accidental neglect is excluded at the misdemeanor level. We should include all individuals who have been convicted of the crime of animal abuse as appropriate for evaluation for a human service intervention. In support of this, currently, statutes in 34 states mandate or at least permit psychological counseling for such individuals.

In addition to these general definitions of animal abuse, in our efforts to identify individuals who have abused animals, it is helpful to be aware of the variety of

Table 2.1 A typology of companion animal abuse

Physical abuse
Active maltreatment
Assault
Burning
Poisoning
Shooting
Mutilation
Drowning
Suffocation
Abandonment
Restriction of movement
Incorrect method of training
Inbreeding
Trapping
Transportation (unprotected, overloaded)
Fireworks
Bestiality
Passive neglect or ignorance
Lack of food and water
Lack of shelter
Lack of necessary veterinary care to alleviate suffering from illness or injury
Lack of sanitation
General neglect (dirty, lack of grooming, poor body condition)
Commercial exploitation
Excessive labor
Fighting
Indiscriminate breeding
Sport (racing)
Experimentation
Mental abuse
Active maltreatment
Instillment of fear, anguish, anxiety
Passive neglect
Deprivation of love and affection

From Vermeulen and Odendaal (1993)

forms of abuse. As does violence directed at humans (e.g., threats, simple assault, aggravated assault, sexual assault, and murder), violence directed at and abuse of animals encompasses many different behaviors. Vermeulen and Odendaal (1993) present a typology divided into physical and mental abuse and further break down the former into active maltreatment, passive neglect or ignorance, and commercial exploitation (Table 2.1). Note that mental or emotional abuse, while recognized statutorily in child abuse, domestic violence, and elder abuse laws, has never been applied to animal anti-cruelty laws in the United States.

Table 2.2 Types of animal abusers

Violent aggressors	Extreme and lethal violence, usually primary intended victim is human
Hapless abusers	Activity, often criminal, in which harm to animal is accidental or incidental
Career abusers	Legal profit making activity involving animal abuse
Disciplinarians	Abusive punishment for disobedience
Schemers and cons	Quasi-business activities involving neglect and abandonment
Thrill seekers	Primarily adolescents acting in groups
Control freaks	Abusive punishment for unrealistic regimen
Racketeers	Illegal profit making activity, such as dog- and cockfighting
Hoarders	Collecting large numbers of animals beyond available resources
Neglectors	Failure to provide adequate food, water, and shelter

Adapted from Bickerstaff (2003)

Based on a study of media reports of alleged anti-cruelty crimes, Bickerstaff found ten individual types of abusers (Table 2.2). These types are a mix of those based on context and purpose of the abuse and motivation of the abuser.

Gerbasi (2004) provides a similarly mixed set of types of abuse based on a sample taken from a web-based listing of media reports (petabuse.com): bestiality, fighting, hoarding, neglect/abandonment, and direct abuse (beating, torturing, or shooting). She found that all types predominantly involve male perpetrators, except hoarding which is predominantly a female behavior.

Another way of categorizing types of abuse is to organize them based on likely etiology. Tedeschi suggests three such categories—crimogenic, traumogenic, and psychogenic (Tedeschi, personal communication, 2015). Crimogenic refers to a history of criminal conduct, particularly involving violence and aggression (fights or bullying). Traumogenic refers to the presence of posttraumatic symptoms such as intense distress or active avoidance of situations that arouse memory of traumatic events. Psychogenic includes indications of serious mental or developmental disorders. As a fourth category, we add envirogenic to refer to non-traumatic familial and/or cultural determinants such as socialization in a dysfunctional family and subcultural norms that model violent and abusive behavior (e.g., dog- and cock fighting).

Finally, the literature on types of human-on-human aggression provides helpful indicators and distinctions applicable in the context of animal abuse. A major distinction is between instrumental and expressive acts of aggression (Downey et al. 2000). Instrumental or predatory aggression is the purposive use of aggression to accomplish a specific goal or a general goal, such as control of another individual. By contrast, expressive or affective aggression involves loss of control occasioned by emotional distress, such as anger, fear, or shame. Predatory aggressors are callous, showing little emotion and positive satisfaction in their violent acts. Expressive aggressors are overly sensitive to other individuals' behavior. They are prone to anxiously expect, distort perception of, and to react violently to perceived rejection (Gupta 2008).

2.2 Sources of Identification of Abuse

In addition to the various professions within the human services, other possible sources of identification of individuals who have abused or are at risk of abusing animals include the criminal justice system, veterinary medicine, and humane education. We discuss these briefly, before turning to policies and practices facilitating identification in the human services.

2.2.1 Criminal Justice System

Enforcement of anti-cruelty laws is the major source of individuals who abuse animals. Depending on the jurisdiction, this may fall under the purview of local law enforcement agencies, humane societies, or SPCAs with no consistent pattern. Once adjudicated and convicted, courts are the major source of referrals of adults. Adults who have been adjudicated on animal cruelty charges, which, as described, could include simple neglect, intentional cruelty, animal hoarding, animal fighting, and sexual assault, may be referred to a mental health professional by the courts for an evaluation and/or treatment. Currently, 34 states either mandate or provide discretionary authority for judges to order counseling for various types of animal abuse (National District Attorney 2015). In 25 cases, judges have specified AniCare as the required form of treatment. (This is an unknown but likely small percentage of cases before the court.)

Given the co-occurrence of human violence and animal abuse, any individual convicted of interpersonal violence may also be abusing animals, or at risk for doing so. In response to this empirical evidence of the link between animal cruelty and domestic violence, 28 states now permit protective orders to include companion animals (Animal Welfare Institute 2015). Several counties and at least one state (Tennessee) have created registries for adults convicted of animal abuse, similar to those for sex offenders; however, utilization and enforcement of these registries have been minimal. Twenty-three states require offenders convicted of bestiality or animal sexual assault to be added to sex offender registries.

The Federal Bureau of Investigation maintains a national crime data base, the National Incident-Based Reporting System (NIBRS), which is comprised of data collected from 18,000 local police agencies throughout the United States (Rajewski 2015). In 2014, four types of animal cruelty and neglect were added as a crime which means that detailed data on reported incidents will be collected and analyzed about animal cruelty crimes, regardless of whether there was an arrest or conviction. The FBI classified animal cruelty as a crime against society, rather than a property crime. The inclusion of these categories involving animal abuse will likely increase investigations by police and the availability of public documents on individual perpetrators. It also will lead to better information on the causes and correlates of animal cruelty, which, in turn, will inform human service efforts to treat this population.

Related to this shift by the FBI, the field of animal law is now part of the curriculum at more than 140 law schools. Many state bar associations have formed sections on animal law. The two national associations of prosecuting attorneys, the Association of Prosecuting Attorneys (APA) and the National District Attorneys Association (NDAA), also provide training to prosecutors and police on animal abuse and its relation to human violence. The NDAA has published a monograph that provides guidelines to the development and prosecution of cases of alleged animal abuse (Phillips and Lockwood 2013). Other national groups, including the National Link Coalition (2015a), also have been involved in training law enforcement, judges, police, mental health professionals, and others on the significance of the association between animal abuse and other crimes.

Taken together, these trends within the criminal justice system provide an expanding process for the identification of individuals who have abused or are at risk for abusing animals.

2.2.2 Veterinary Medicine

Like many personnel in the criminal justice system, veterinarians are positioned to be "first responders" or, more aptly here, first points of contact in instances of animal abuse, similar to physicians as first responders to child abuse and domestic violence (Arkow and Munro 2008). Through a combination of available screening instruments and clinical judgment, veterinarians can be alert to medical conditions that are attributable to animal abuse.

The description of a "battered pet" syndrome by Munro (1996), similar to long-established protocols for battered children and women, initiated a veterinary perspective on the recognition and reporting of suspected animal abuse. The Tufts Animal Care and Condition scales provide visual guidelines for assessing body condition, physical care, environmental safety, and sanitation (Patronek 1997). Neglectful behavior is often immediately evident (e.g., emaciation, severely matted hair). Intentionally abusive and violent behavior must be distinguished from accidental injury (e.g., car accident). An extensive literature of veterinary forensics and veterinary pathology materials and training materials describe client behaviors and presenting clinical conditions that should arouse suspicion of abuse (e.g., burns, poisoning, gunshot wounds, head injuries, rib fracture, blunt force injury; Miller and Zawistowski 1997).

Once having identified animal abuse or risk of it, the possible and responsible actions of veterinarians are complex, involving legal, financial, peer, professional, practice management, and ethical issues (Arkow et al. 2011). While these are largely beyond the purview of human service providers, it is helpful to be aware of the issues for, as we will describe, comparable issues arise in human service contexts. Patronek (1997) discusses documentation to assure systematic and rigorous evidence gathering which may be helpful in the case of prosecution. Reporting to legal authorities raises issues of confidentiality to the client (in the veterinary context, the caretaker) as against the welfare of the animal and, given the association between human violence and animal abuse, the safety of the human community. Currently, veterinarians in 15 states are mandated and in 5 states are permitted to report animal abuse.

After legal obligations to report are met, veterinarians have the option of referral to an appropriate human service agency (Arkow et al. 2011). Many localities have formed coalitions of stakeholders based on a common concern with reducing violence whether toward humans or other animals (National Link Coalition 2015a). These coalitions provide networking between veterinary, criminal justice, animal welfare, and human service personnel, among others.

Through the emerging field of veterinary social work, social work departments partner with veterinary schools to educate veterinary students in issues such as grief and companion animal loss, the link between human and animal violence, animal-assisted interactions, and compassion fatigue (Arkow 2015a).

2.2.3   Public Education

The public is one source of identification and reporting of animal abuse. Not surprisingly, public concern about animal welfare is lower than that found in the animal protection movement (Taylor and Signal 2006a, b). In another study, Taylor and Signal (pp. 201–211) found a number of factors associated with a greater propensity to report animal abuse by members of the general public: gender (female), occupation (nonanimal related), and acknowledgment of the link between human violence and animal abuse.

The animal protection movement, including animal workers in shelters and sanctuaries, can be both a source of identification and reporting and, as well, a source of public education. Humane education as a field has grown significantly in recent years. While traditionally largely limited to instruction in responsible care for companion animals, increasingly the curriculum includes discussion of animal abuse and its relationship to other crime, as well as environmental issues (Weil 2004). In the context of primary prevention, humane education is being integrated into social and emotional learning for children as a way to prevent and sometimes discover the occurrence of violence against animals and people. Red Rover Readers is a humane literacy program that aims to foster empathy and compassion in children while teaching literacy skills (Red Rover 2015).

2.2.4   Human Services

As we have indicated, given its association with human violence and criminality generally, animal abuse is a social as well as an animal welfare problem. However, it is likely that most animal abuse still goes unidentified or, if identified, is not appropriately addressed. While aided by the increased efforts of the institutions and agencies discussed above, human service agencies and practitioners are ideally positioned to rectify this shortcoming.

In most human service settings, providers can and should include an inquiry about the presence and welfare of companion animals in clients' current living situation and family history. Since doing so often facilitates the building of rapport and disclosure generally, providers should make this inquiry in the initial contact. Whether the context is an intake, referral, assessment, or intervention, we strongly suggest that providers adopt the mantra, "always ask" about animal abuse. In response to a query about their current living situation and interpersonal relationships, if clients do not mention the presence of animals, it is expedient to ask, "Are there any animals in or at the home?" or "Does your girlfriend have a companion animal?" Once the presence of animals is established, inquiry should proceed to an eventual query about animal abuse. However, questioning should begin with items less likely to provoke defensive responses: "Has a companion animal of yours ever been hurt; have you ever seen anyone hurt a companion animal; have you ever hurt a companion animal?" We provide a more detailed and structured version of a screening device adapted from Boat (1999; Sect. 4.2).

While we advise always asking, human service providers working with certain populations are more likely to encounter clients who have abused or are at risk for abusing animals and should be especially disposed to include inquiry about that possibility. At this relatively early period in the effort by human services to address the problem of animal abuse, the literature on the diagnoses and comorbid conditions of people who abuse animals is limited but growing. As discussed, an exception is the inclusion of cruelty to animals as an indicator of Conduct Disorder of Childhood (American Psychiatric Association 1987) and its relationship to the adult diagnosis of Antisocial Personality Disorder. Clearly, individuals so diagnosed should be carefully assessed for the presence of animal abuse.

Notwithstanding the need for direct diagnostic studies of animal abusers, the literature on populations in which animal abuse commonly co-occurs is instructive, particularly that on perpetrators of interpersonal violence (IPV). "[T]he vast majority of perpetrators [of domestic violence] suffer from one or more conditions, including affective disorders, personality disorders, neurological disorders, trauma-related disorders, and psychoactive substance disorders" (Sonkin and Liebert 2003, p. 7). In a study that included victims as well as perpetrators of IPV, Stuart et al. (2006) found that alcohol problems in perpetrators and their partners contributed directly to physical abuse and indirectly to psychological aggression. Finally, George et al. (2006) add "…diagnoses related to anxiety, depression, intermittent explosive disorder, and borderline personality disorder" (p. 345) in a population of domestic violence perpetrators.

Given these findings, human service workers working with individuals who present with issues involving IPV, other criminal activity, substance abuse, personality disorders, and, to some extent, anxiety and depression should thoroughly screen for animal abuse.

Another important source of the identification of animal abuse, largely although not entirely within human services, is cross-reporting and cross-training. Given the link between human violence and animal abuse, the presence of one is an indicator of the possible presence of the other. Personnel working in the area of domestic violence, for example, should be trained to identify and report to providers and agencies trained to work with the assessment and treatment of animal abuse. At present, such cross-reporting and cross-training are limited to providers working with children.

Currently, four states mandate and eight permit child agencies to report animal abuse. In the other direction, nine states mandate animal agencies to report child abuse. Only three states (Connecticut, Illinois, and West Virginia) mandate full two-way cross-reporting between child and animal protection agencies, but enforcement and effectiveness of this are unknown (National Link Coalition 2015b). We discuss professional ethical and legal issues raised by cross-reporting below under the subheading "Confidentiality" (pp. 37–39).

2.3   Assessment

2.3.1   Introduction

Once having identified the presence or risk of animal abuse, we can move to assessment proper. How are we to determine diagnosis, formulation, form of intervention, and, if necessary, appropriate referral? At this relatively early stage in the recognition of the need for intervention for this population, there are few, if any, validated assessment instruments (Ascione and Shapiro 2009, p. 571). Some more generic inventories do include one relevant item but that is limited to establishing the presence or absence of animal abuse. In recent years, researchers have developed instruments designed to measure animal abuse and characterize individuals who abuse animals; however, they are limited to childhood and adolescent populations. For a critical review, see Ascione and Shapiro (2009, p. 571–573).

Given the high incidence of reports of animal abuse (Luke et al. 1997), including a number that are court-ordered cases, and the co-occurrence of animal abuse with violence toward humans, it is incumbent on us to provide the best available assessment instruments and interventions. These must be continually informed by our growing experience of working with this population and forthcoming research.

Rather than validated instruments, then, in this section on assessment, we provide tools that have the more modest goal of facilitating the development of a socio-psychological *portrait* of clients who abuse animals. Given the several forms of animal abuse and the various pathways to animal abuse, we expect to find that it has many different faces. The portraits can then be used to guide the development of a course of action, whether that is specification of a treatment plan within the present agency, referral to another human service agency, or, in high-risk cases, to a criminal justice agency.

We suggest that the primary vehicle for the development of the portrait is the use of semi-structured interviews. Existing checklists that identify and evaluate factors such as form and extent of animal abuse, motives, conflict areas, interpersonal dynamics, and preconditions can guide these interviews. We will present below a checklist that amalgamates several existing surveys in the literature. In addition, the screening device in Sect. 4.2 and the extensive psychological and social history instrument in Sect. 4.3 may be helpful in developing a full picture of the client. It is also important to assess for existing primary and/or comorbid conditions, as well as conditions known to be co-occurring with animal abuse.

2.3.2   Assessment for Comorbid and/or Co-occurring Disorders

While formal research on the issue is sorely needed, from our experience with the earlier edition of AniCare with adults and from anecdotal evidence of individual cases, it is apparent that there are many pathways to and comorbid presentations associated with the behavior of animal abuse. Individuals can suffer from any one of the following disorders listed in the current diagnostic manual (American Psychiatric Association 2013): schizophrenia spectrum, bipolar, depressive, anxiety, trauma, obsessive-compulsive, sexual dysfunction, impulse-control, conduct, dissociative, substance-related disorders, or personality disorders. When the history, the initial interaction, or a simple mental status examination suggest the presence of a particular disorder, human service providers can use those instruments customarily employed in their practice or agency at intake or when making a referral to establish the presence of these conditions.

As discussed earlier in the context of identification, the co-occurrence of IPV, other criminal activity, and animal abuse suggests that providers be especially alert to the possible presence of these disorders in individuals identified as having abused animals. In addition to taking a history of IPV and other criminal activity and recourse to public records, providers can employ relevant assessment tools. The Personality Assessment Inventory, a general or broad-based instrument, is particularly useful for assessing disorders involving antisocial behavior such as antisocial personality, oppositional defiant, and conduct disorders (Douglas et al. 2001).

2.3.3   Specific Assessment of Animal Abuse

The Checklist of Factors in the Assessment of Animal Abuse (hereafter, checklist) is an adaptation and amalgamation of several existing surveys (Table 2.3). Many of the factors or variables found in individuals who have abused animals have clear counterparts in abusive human-human interactions. For example, the need to control and dominate may take different behavioral forms but often is underlying in both contexts. Some factors have analogs in the human-human context, but arguably assume a distinct form in the animal context. For example, speciesism, discrimination against an individual based on species difference, is analogous to but distinct from sexism and racism. In a given individual, some factors may generalize to human-human relationships; others may be confined to human-animal contexts. For example, an individual may externalize blame across the board but only have a prejudice against or scapegoat animals or even one species of animal.

The subsections below provide elaboration of selected items in each of the major subheads of the checklist.

2.3.3.1 Severity

This subsection focuses on the abusive behavior itself and its impact on the animal victims. Single instances of animal abuse, unless egregious, are not as significant psychologically as recurring abuse (Hensley et al. 2012), as the latter shows an

Table 2.3 Checklist of factors in the assessment of animal abuse

Severity
Degree of injury (mild, moderate, severe)
Frequency and duration (how many times, over what span of time)
Number and kind of species, including level of sentience (degree that an animal is capable of sensation or feeling)
Prolonged or immediate
Intimacy of infliction of injury (compare whether stabbed or shot at distance)
Culpability
Capable of understanding consequences
Knowledge of what constitutes a criminal act
Awareness of extent of animal suffering
Refusal to accept responsibility for the abuse
Refusal to accept that abuse is wrong
Subculture or family sanction of the abuse of animals
Resistance to assessment
Externalizing of blame
Degree of planning
Obstacles that were overcome
Alone or in a group: if in group, leader or follower
Coercion by a more dominant individual
Motivation/psychodynamics
Curiosity/experimentation
Reaction to fear of animal
Approval of others
Peer pressure (culture of hyper-masculinity)
Coercion of or retaliation against a human
Reaction to personal experience of abuse/punishment (posttraumatic attempt for mastery/control; identification with the aggressor; displacement of aggression)
Lack of positive interactions with animal (instability of relationships)
Mood enhancement (relief from boredom or depression)
Alleviation of feelings of powerlessness, loneliness, or alienation
Rehearsal or enhancement of one's own aggressiveness
Hypersensitivity to real or perceived threats
Narcissistic slights/rage
Other antisocial behavior (aggression in family, with peers, or strangers; property crime; drug-related offenses)
Pleasure from inflicting suffering (sadism)
Sexual assault of an animal and/or sexual arousal resulting from abuse
Documented abuse with video or photograph and/or returned to scene to relive
Ritualistic features

(continued)

Table 2.3 (continued)

Attitudes/beliefs
Unaware of the physical and psychological needs of animals and different species
Belief that animals exist for instrumental purposes only
Little or no thought to the roles and positions of animals in human society
Prejudice against a particular species (e.g., cats)
Cruelty as a way to control and "discipline" an animal
Cultural practice or acceptance of abusive behavior
Emotional intelligence
Capacity for empathy
Capacity to form a secure relationship
Capable of reciprocal relationship
Understanding of relationships (reciprocation, accommodation)
Capable of forming attachments
Openness to change
Family history
Domestic violence
Physical, emotional, or sexual abuse as child
Physical or emotional neglect
Animal abuse
Relationships with animals
Harsh and inconsistent discipline
Spanking and other physical punishment
Mitigating circumstances
Acceptance of responsibility
Expression of feelings of remorse, shame, or guilt
Seeking to make restitution
Assistance to law enforcement
Capable of forming bond with an animal
Understanding of motives for the abuse

The Checklist was derived from a variety of sources, including Arluke (1997); Ascione (2001); Ascione et al. (1997); Boat (1999); Jory and Randour (1998); Kellert and Felthous (1985); Lewchanin and Zimmerman (2000); Lockwood (1998), and Colorado Link Project (2015) established pattern of behavior. As discussed, although the degree of injury and suffering may be greater, neglectful behavior implies less serious or at least different problems than does intentional abuse. "Prolonged" or "immediate" refers to the duration of a given instance of abuse. Both it and "intimacy of infliction of injury" address perpetrators' comfort with or need to be "up close and personal" with their victims and imply more serious and likely recalcitrant problems.

2.3.3.2 Culpability

To what extent do clients accept responsibility for the abuse? Lack of acceptance may be based on the belief that animals do not have the capacity to suffer or that their suffering is not an ethical issue and that, therefore, they did not do anything wrong. Other clients may not have sufficient intelligence to understand the consequences of the abuse, either from the point view of the animal suffering or the criminality involved. They should be referred for an appropriate intervention.

Abuse that involves planning and overcoming obstacles to affect the abuse indicates adequate intelligence, and, likely, some deliberation about consequences usually implies culpability. By contrast, clients that abuse animals on impulse are unlikely to have considered consequences.

Clients acting in groups often deny culpability claiming that they were responding to peer pressure, didn't know of the intent to abuse, or felt intimidated by a strong leader. It is important to determine whether clients were leaders or followers.

Assessment of culpability is an important issue in the development of a working therapeutic relationship as refusal to accept any responsibility that can be part of a refusal to admit the need for counseling. We discuss ways to establish accountability below as part of the initial phase of therapy. It is important to assess the degree and basis of resistance to accepting responsibility. In some clients, the resistance is situational, while in others it is part of a general trait (e.g., externalizing blame or defensiveness).

2.3.3.3 Motivation/Psychodynamics

In general, it is important to distinguish abuse in which animals are the direct object of hostility or anger from cases in which it is displaced aggression or an instrument to control, intimidate, or retaliate against humans. When animals are the actual object, distinguish further between frustration resulting from failure to control an animal from reaction out of fear of an animal. Also, distinguish these latter reasons from prejudice against a species of animals.

The items under this subheading are listed *roughly* from the more psychologically benign to the more problematic and/or resistant to change.

- It is common in normal development for a child to "experiment" with animals (often limited to insects). If this practice extends into adolescence and early adulthood, it is more serious. In any case, some intervention should be recommended (e.g., education or psychoeducation).

- A fear reaction is unlikely to be premeditated and can be largely in the context of a response of self-defense. Directly socially mediated abuse (approval of others; peer pressure) often occurs in the context of a subculture of hyper-masculinity and devalues any empathic concern about the animal victims. Like the experimentation item, this is more serious when occurring in late adolescence or early adulthood.
- Individuals motivated to coerce or retaliate against another human are using the animal victim as an instrument and the animal is not the primary object of the violence.
- If an aggressive reaction to a personal experience of abuse in childhood is still operative in adult clients, it may have become a habitual and primary way of solving problems in living.
- Mood enhancement is a common motive in adolescence (boredom). In adulthood, if in response to depressive feelings, it may be part of a depressive disorder.
- Clients who abuse animals to relieve negative feelings such as loneliness or alienation may be dealing with unresolved dependent needs which, being unfulfilled by an animal, result in frustration and abuse.
- Many serial killers rehearsed or practiced on animals before turning to human victims.
- Hypersensitivity to threats may imply misattribution of the motives of animals and can be part of a paranoid stance.
- Narcissistically based abuse suggests overidentification with an animal and is common in the context of dog fighting when a dog does not live up to the self-image of the person.
- Other antisocial behavior, sadism, sexual assault, and documentation of the abuse by the perpetrator (e.g., filming it) are, of course, indicative of a serious psychological disorder. Abuse in the context of ritualistic practices is embedded in a subculture and is likely to be highly resistant to change.

2.3.3.4 Attitudes/Beliefs

These are ingrained views of animals that may have originated in the subculture or family of origin, or may reflect personality traits (e.g., narcissistic or paranoid). Whether made explicit or not, we all have to answer questions about the nature of and the proper attitudes toward other animals: is an animal a sentient being, a thing, a property item, a member of the family, someone with whom I may have a relationship, a resource or an instrument, or an appropriate object of moral consideration? Given the many distinctions we make among the animals that surround us (companion, farmed, wild, feral, zoo, and laboratory), these more general attitudes often apply to some categories but not others (pigs are for eating, dogs for company, deer for hunting).

2.3.3.5 Emotional Intelligence

As in any assessment, it is important to evaluate clients' strengths as well as their deficits. These positive personality features should be assessed in both human-human and human-animal contexts as they may be evident in only one of these. Does a client have the ability to form attachments that are relatively secure? Prior attachments to companion animals are a common experience of people who then abuse them. See attachment theory discussion (pp. 62–63, 99–100). Some clients may have the capacity for empathy, but have learned not to empathize with animals (or with animals of a particular species, such as cats). See Sect. 3.3.2 for a more detailed discussion of the assessment of the important skill of empathy. It is critical to take a history of clients' relationships with animals and to identify instances of positive or at least ambivalent relationships with an animal, as well as abusive relationships.

2.3.3.6 Family History

For this population of adults who have abused animals, providers should give special attention to a history of domestic violence and animal abuse both in clients' family of origin and in their current living situation. Also, given the possible role of trauma as a precursor to animal abuse, a history of childhood abuse and neglect should be included. An assessment of the form of discipline that clients' experienced in childhood is important as there is evidence that physical punishment by fathers may be a precursor of animal abuse (Flynn 1999). We have included a generic psychological/ sociological survey that may be used as a resource (Sect. 4.3). It includes a violent behavior checklist and questions about legal history.

2.3.3.7 Mitigating Circumstances

Clients' responses to the fact of their abuse of animals are important indicators of their willingness and ability to deal with the problem constructively and cooperatively in both counseling and criminal justice settings.

2.3.4 Risk Assessment

While many of the issues already discussed in this section on assessment are likely risk factors, here we give special attention to risk assessment as the target behavior of animal abuse, which can require immediate precautionary intervention to protect the welfare of both animals and humans.

But first a critical note about risk assessment is in order. Our ability to predict violent behavior toward humans with respect to an individual is limited (Gupta 2008, p. 224). Even with respect to groups of individuals, at best we can assign a higher probability of the occurrence of the behavior for high-risk as compared to low-risk populations. Researchers distinguish between risk assessment as an attempt to predict violent behavior and "threat assessment," which more modestly attempts to prevent violence by "interrupt[ing] people on a pathway to commit [violence]" (Miller 2014, p. 38). Webster (Forensic Psychiatry.ca 2015) provides a listing and critique of available risk assessment instruments for general human violence, spousal assault, and sexual violence.

Currently, there are no risk-validated assessment instruments that effectively identify potential perpetrators of animal abuse, and the literature on risk or threat assessment generally does not include animal abuse as an indicator. However, the empirical association of violence toward humans and animal abuse justifies the conservative use of existing risk assessment instruments targeting the general population of violent offenders. Conversely, the presence of animal abuse should be considered as a risk factor for human violence as well as future animal abuse. These considerations should be part of any assessment as they can indicate the choice of intervention—for example, crisis intervention or placement in a diversion program.

In addition to a history of animal abuse or human violence, what should we consider as possible risk or threat precursors to future occurrences of either of these behaviors? Some indicators are risk factors for many different presenting conditions: demographics such as age and gender; general factors such as anxiety, depression, and insecure attachments; past behaviors such as other criminal acts, sexual assault, and substance abuse; and situational factors such as loss, failure, or public humiliation. However, studies suggest that the following may be more directly linked to animal abuse:

- Fire setting (Becker et al. 2004)
- Corporal punishment (Flynn 1999)
- Exposure to domestic violence (Henry 2004)
- Witnessing animal abuse (Gullone and Robertson 2008)
- Callousness or sensitivity to rejection (Gupta 2008)
- Low caregiving (Henry 2006)

Assessors should consider both these direct indicators and the more general or indirect indicators in the context of the entire assessment, including positive or protective factors such as those listed in the Mitigating Circumstances section of the checklist (p. 28).

Risk and threat assessment instruments were largely developed and are currently used in the criminal justice system to prevent criminal activity by identifying individuals likely to commit violent acts. In the context of human services, practitioners have the responsibility of assessing risk and reporting high-risk individuals to the appropriate criminal justice authorities. We address the question of a "duty to report" and related professional legal and ethical issues below under the sub heading "Confidentiality" (pp. 37–39).

Assessment that identifies individuals at risk of future animal abuse is also useful within the treatment context as it is relevant to the form of treatment recommended. When individuals are judged to be at high risk for imminent animal abuse—whether in an assessment or an ongoing treatment context, crisis intervention should be considered. This might involve notifying caretakers of companion animals in the family of the client of imminent risk to the animals or to themselves.

For individuals at medium risk, a diversionary program might be recommended, where indicated, supplemented by individual counseling. These are individuals for whom there is long term but little immediate risk of abusive behavior. They might include those with no history of or a single instance of animal abuse.

For individuals at low risk, if the court does not prohibit it, therapists should consider limiting clients' contact with animals outside of the session and cautious use of animals in the therapy.

2.3.5 Treatment Options

Many clients are court ordered for assessment and treatment of animal abuse; in effect, that is their "presenting problem." However, for these and most other clients, animal abuse is part of a larger set of problems. A major issue in recommending a treatment plan is whether the intervention should address the behavior of animal abuse as the primary or as a secondary problem. Put another way, should animal abuse be treated as a symptom of other problems or as the primary target behavior of the treatment? To some extent, providers answer these questions according to their general approach to therapy. Cognitive behaviorists focus on the presenting target behavior; psychodynamically oriented therapists take the presenting problem as symptomatic of an underlying disorder; and experience-based therapists largely follow the direction of their clients. Answers also are influenced by the fact that court orders may specify elimination of animal abuse as the purpose of the intervention and support only a limited number of sessions which circumscribe the forms of intervention. Finally, as discussed, treatment, at least initially, may be dictated by high risk of harm to others, human or animal. Obviously, our bottom-line concern should be to make treatment recommendations tailored to the individual client based on a thorough assessment.

A related issue is whether the treatment of animal abuse can be assimilated into the broader current practices of human service providers or requires interventions unique to that behavior. In this early stage of the development of the AniCare approach as an evidence-based practice, we leave this as an open question for individual providers to answer. We would think that answers will be a function of the primacy of animal abuse as the presenting problem and of providers' approach to therapy. While in this text we often refer to the "AniCare approach," implying that it is a stand-alone and unique set of interventions, providers are free to borrow and adapt components of the intervention as needed. In such cases, AniCare offers a toolbox rather than a general approach.

In terms of the framework of primary, secondary, and tertiary prevention discussed in the context of violence connection policy, most clients who reach the stage of having a full assessment will require some form of tertiary intervention. However, in some instances, secondary interventions may be helpful, particularly as complements to tertiary intervention. Diversion programs in group settings that offer training in interpersonal skills, including empathy, education, and value clarification regarding relationships to animals, have been developed for children and could be adapted for adults. Children and Animals Together (CAT; Arizona State University 2015) is a child-centered family intervention that includes assessment, diversion program, and therapy components.

Some court-ordered sentences of individuals convicted of animal abuse raise questions about their appropriateness. Courts commonly require community service that exposes individuals to settings with animals (such as an animal shelter), while, ironically, other courts restrict exposure to animals for a certain period. Based on an assessment, the former may be counterindicated for some if not most clients and, if not properly supervised, puts animals at risk. Courts also sometimes specify anger management as a required intervention. While management of anger and emotional reactivity more generally may be problems for some individuals in this varied population, the assessment should determine the appropriate intervention on a case-by-case basis. Evaluators and providers should be mindful of the need to educate criminal justice personnel about the varied needs of this population.

Assessors can choose recommended treatment from a broad spectrum of options. For a general discussion of options, see The Colorado Link Project website, (2015). In terms of the intensity of intervention, we locate AniCare near the middle of that spectrum. At the less intensive end, we have discussed diversion programs, anger, and emotional reactivity management and, at least in terms of duration of the intervention, crisis intervention. Another form of less intensive treatment, psychoeducation, involves teaching clients about and sensitizing them to psychological issues, such as identifying feelings and developing interpersonal skills. In this context, psycho-education could focus on recognizing the needs and interests of animals and learning appropriate human-animal interaction.

At the more intensive end, in-patient or residential treatment may be appropriate for clients diagnosed with major affective, schizophrenic spectrum disorders, and severe cases of personality disorders such as borderline personality. Where possible, components of the residential treatment can use specific exercises from AniCare to address the specific behavior of animal abuse. Psychiatric treatment or intensive psychological treatment complemented by a psychopharmacological regimen may be indicated for such cases—again, supplemented by special attention to the problem of animal abuse. In some such cases, animal-assisted therapy may be helpful, with appropriate precautions taken for the welfare of the animals involved.

Intensive or at least labor-intensive interventions may be necessary for clients evaluated to be lacking skills in daily living—for example, self-neglect and inadequate personal care. In such cases, referral to caseworkers skilled in using community resources to help manage clients may be indicated. In cases where the underlying problem is dysfunctional, human-human relationships and abuse of animals have largely an instrumental function, marriage or family therapy might be the treatment of choice. A comorbid disorder such as substance abuse may require treatment before clients can address the problem of animal abuse.

The place of AniCare in this array of treatment options varies. In cases where less intensive interventions would be inadequate and more intensive interventions are not necessary, AniCare can be the sole intervention. As discussed, in our experience, most clients who have abused animals present with other problems as well. However, these complexities often involve sociological and environmental issues rather than the presence of a diagnosable disorder—chronically unsatisfactory interpersonal relationships, unemployment, and poor health. In these cases, the

AniCare treatment is appropriate, supplemented where necessary by resources provided by other social agencies.

When AniCare is the sole intervention, providers can be advised to emphasize different components of the approach—as we will describe further in the Treatment section. For example, clients whose animal abuse is a form of instrumental or predatory aggression may benefit from emphasis on empathic skills while other interpersonal skills may be more effective with those whose abuse is expressive or affective aggression.

Regarding instances where a combination of treatment approaches are indicated, assessors can be guided by the relative prominence of the animal abuse problem. Where more prominent, AniCare should be the main intervention supplemented by others, and, conversely, where less prominent, tools from AniCare should be supplemental. Recommendations for mixed treatments can also specify the order of interventions. Treatment of substance abuse should precede treatment of the animal abuse; couples or family therapy should follow treatment for animal abuse.

Late adolescent clients may benefit from a combination of interventions in AniCare Child and AniCare Adult. For example, some such clients have very limited vocabularies of and access to their feelings (Shapiro et al. 2014, pp. 25–28).

Intervention

3

3.1 The Initial Phase of Therapy: Establishing a Working Relationship

3.1.1 Joining the Client

Depending on theoretical bent, target populations treated, and personal style, therapists develop their own ways of joining, connecting, or establishing a working alliance with their clients. Common tactics involve adopting the clients' language, using candid language or straight talk, acknowledging a personal interest of the client (vocational or avocational), empathizing with the clients' feelings, and exploring the clients' views of the therapy and therapist. See Shapiro et al. (2014, pp. 26–30) for discussion of this initial phase of therapy in working with children. Clients' views of the therapy are particularly important when working with adult clients who abuse animals as they often are court ordered to be in counseling. In addition to exploring the clients' feelings ("I didn't do anything wrong," "I really don't have time for this," "I am just here 'cause the judge told me to come"), the therapist at the outset needs to clarify his or her own relation to the court. Understandably, the client is concerned that the therapist is at best wearing two hats, one as agent of the court and another as human service provider—"Who are you working for, anyway?" To begin to gain the trust of the client, the therapist needs to acknowledge the issue that the therapy is court ordered as he or she and the client negotiate goals of the therapy (see discussion in "True Intentions" exercise below, p. 34). The issue also colors and complicates the problem of client accountability which presents another block to establishing a working relation—discussed immediately below.

The influence of the involuntary nature of these clients' participation in the therapy cannot be overstated, and the therapist should assume that it is a consideration for the client in all phases of the therapy. Some clients will persist in presenting what they think the judge or prosecutor wants to hear, while others, even more problematically for the therapy, will severely limit what they disclose.

© Springer International Publishing Switzerland 2016
K. Shapiro, A.J.Z. Henderson, *The Identification, Assessment, and Treatment of Adults Who Abuse Animals: The AniCare Approach*,
DOI 10.1007/978-3-319-27362-4_3

3.1.2 "Countertransference": Therapist Feelings Toward the Client

An ongoing task for the therapist is dealing with his or her own feelings toward the client. When working with clients whose actions are socially unacceptable and/or morally offensive, this is particularly challenging. As therapists working with adults who abuse animals often self-select because of their love of animals, therapists working with this population face a very real occupational hazard. The challenge is greatest in the first sessions when the client is typically telling the story of the abusive interactions with animals that are the occasion of them being in therapy. It is also most critical at this time as it can negatively impact the establishment of a good working therapist-client relationship. These feelings can be strong and readily available to the therapist, or they can be more subtle and not fully in his or her awareness.

> For an example of tensions between a therapist and his client in an initial session and, arguably, of therapist feelings coloring the interaction, see Demonstration DVD, Clinical Exercises submenu, Clinical Exercise #2. See Sect. 4.1 for a brief description of this client—"John."

In the literature on psychoanalytic and psychodynamic therapy, dealing with those feelings toward the client that are unconscious and projected from earlier unresolved issues ("countertransference") is a critical task for the therapist. More generally, any emotional response to the client's abuse of animals is a problem to which the therapist must attend.

Therapists can avail themselves of a number of ways of dealing with these feelings. At the extreme, the client can be referred to another therapist. However, our experience with attendees of AniCare workshops suggests that most providers can work out any negative feelings toward these clients within the therapy, in some cases with one or two consultations with a colleague or supervisor. Once they are worked through or, in some instances, as a way to work them through, the therapist can bring the feelings into the therapy in a strategic fashion. For example, the therapist, through inquiry, can establish that the client's behavior and/or attitudes toward animals arouse the same negative feelings in other people: "It makes me feel uncomfortable when you say that. Do you think it may make other people around you uncomfortable? Were you aware of that? Can you become aware of it?" (Shapiro et al. 2014, p. 20).

Another strategy that therapists may use when dealing with their own reactions to the client's abusive behavior is to focus on an underlying feeling, such as shame, guilt, or anxiety, thereby bypassing the offending behavior. This allows the therapist to label the behavior in a way that indirectly confirms his or her negative feelings: "I can understand that it is embarrassing (distressing, disturbing…) for you to talk about (own, accept…) what you did to those animals." This intervention presumes that the client admits to or is at least ambivalent about the acceptability of the behavior and accepts responsibility for it—as we have discussed and will discuss further under this heading, a condition that often does not occur. By redirecting and reflecting on a more socially acceptable underlying feeling, the therapist takes the direct focus of the therapy, for the moment, away from the offensive behavior. Also, by joining the client, he or she may help the relationship.

Animal-assisted therapy can be a part of the treatment of adults who abuse animals—as we will discuss more fully below (see Sect. 3.3.7). For some client populations, the presence of a nonhuman animal can reduce concern about countertransference as it provides therapist's emotional distance between therapist and client. However, for the present population, it is often counter-indicated in the early phases of the therapy. The client's behavior with nonhuman animals is obviously an emotionally laden issue. For the resistant and defensive client, it is also a potentially contentious issue.

3.1.3 Framing the Therapy

There are several components to framing the therapy—the rules of the therapy for client and therapist that describe how they will work together. The inclusion of some of these components is different according to the therapist's theoretical bent. Here we focus on those components that are typically either critical to or problematic in working with the several subpopulations of clients who abuse animals—goals, confidentiality, and honesty.

Goals
Goals of counseling mandated by a court may be defined both in time (e.g., 10–12 sessions) and scope (prevention of future abusive animal behavior). Some therapists vary in their comfort with setting explicit goals and with limiting those goals to specific behaviors. However, in working with adults who have abused animals, we advise setting specific behavioral goals in the form of a negotiated contract and recommend the following exercise to that end.

Exercise: True Intentions
A word about the use of the several exercises interspersed throughout this text: Their use generally requires an active and directive approach and, with the exception of the first two exercises presented, assumes a working relationship with the client. In content, most are familiar as variations of interventions in a cognitive-behaviorist approach adapted for the problem of animal abuse. However, several of them are adapted from Jory's Intimate Justice approach to working with clients presenting with the problem of domestic abuse (Jory and Anderson 1999). Many focus on a particular interpersonal skill, again, with the exception of the first two exercises which come within the initial framing phase of the therapy.

Many, if not most, animal abusers enter therapy under court order. Some attend to avoid probation or jail or to make a positive impression on a judge. For others, the courts have stipulated counseling. Some adolescents are required to attend by their parents. Most of these clients enter therapy feeling that they have been unfairly treated. When clients feel "misunderstood," they begin therapy with little intention of cooperating and may be invested in sabotaging the therapy process. Yet for therapy to be effective, the client needs to be as forthcoming as he or she can be, and in turn, the therapist is obligated to listen with respect and help the client with his or her problems.

The purpose of this exercise is to facilitate the client's eventual adoption of goals in the therapy that minimize the likelihood of future animal abuse. The first move is to invite the client to talk about his or her motives for beginning therapy: "Sometimes it is hard to be honest about what we really want out of therapy. But it will be easier if we discuss honestly what you are hoping for. What are your true intentions for coming to therapy?"

It should not surprise the therapist if the client's motives are primarily self-serving. Self-serving intentions might include "getting out of trouble with the law" or "getting my family off my back." Rather than challenging these, the therapist acknowledges that it is not wrong to be self-serving:

> Those are your goals, your true intentions, and I accept them and appreciate your being straight with me. We will be straight with each other here. I will be honest with you about what mine are and you be honest about what yours are and we will work together.

To challenge clients to be honest with themselves and to coax any hidden agendas into the open (Jory and Anderson 1999, p. 358), the therapist can make non-threatening and open-ended inquiries: "You don't need to change your reasons for coming to therapy, but can we find some other things that you would also agree to work on? Are you willing to consider changing anything about yourself? Do you want to understand animals better? Are you worried that maybe you really have done something wrong?"

Clinical Case

This exchange is adapted from an interview in the Demonstration DVD, Clinical Exercises submenu, Clinical Exercise #3. See Sect. 4.1 for a brief description of this client—"Roy."

Therapist: So this is an important time together. It is a time to learn something about what happened to you, about what you've done – a time to learn something about yourself. But I understand you have your own reasons for coming here. What are your true intentions for being here?

Roy: The parole officer told me to come so I'm here to keep out of jail.

Therapist: I understand that and I appreciate that you are being honest – that you don't want to go back to jail – that you want to do the right thing so you don't have to go back to jail. So inside you, those are your true intentions – something you really want to accomplish. What other things do you want to get out of these sessions?

Roy: That's it. That's all. The court says you got to go to these sessions and I am here.

Therapist: OK, I understand that. But the idea that you might learn something about yourself and learn not to let this happen again – new ideas about your relationships with people and animals—is that totally foreign to you?

Roy: You do what you do and I'll do what I do and we'll see what happens.

Therapist: OK, as we go along, we'll be clear about what you are trying to accomplish and what I am trying to accomplish for you – your true intentions and mine. I'll be honest and straightforward with you about what I think we need to accomplish.

Homework Assignment

Ask the client to list the goals he or she would like to accomplish in therapy. Like most *AniCare* exercises, this works best if the assignment begins in therapy and is then taken home to be worked on. It is usually best if the client writes down these goals and shares them with the therapist because this process brings accountability into play. The list of goals should be available throughout the duration of therapy, so that the therapist and the client can review it together at various points in treatment to see how the client's new intentions compare to his or her original ones.

Confidentiality

Counselor confidentiality or the client-counselor privilege is designed to allow clients the freedom to share private information in an open and safe setting. The presumption is that therapists should always protect client confidentiality unless there is a compelling reason to do otherwise. Defining the extent and limits of confidentiality is requisite to gaining the trust of the client and, therefore, to the establishment and maintenance of an effective, working therapist-client relationship. It is also an important issue in legislation and professional codes of ethics related to therapist conduct.

Two issues arise that are inherent to working with this population. As we have indicated, most cases are court ordered. For the most part, courts recognize that what transpires in the counseling sessions is protected and only requires information such as the number of sessions attended and recommendation as to satisfactory completion or need for further treatment. In rare circumstances, a counselor may be presented with a subpoena that demands the turnover of more substantive information from a client's sessions.

A second issue, the "duty to warn," is more problematic and requires some background discussion. Consider the possibility that the client in the course of the therapy indicates or even suggests the intention to kill or seriously harm an animal. Under what conditions can the therapist break confidence with the client and report this intention to the relevant parties?

While there are strong policies in place that protect therapist-client confidence, there are also exceptions that limit it. In the aftermath of the Tarasoff case (Herbert and Young 2002), the courts upheld and most states have since legislated that therapists have an obligation to warn relevant parties that a client is a "threat to self or others." This "dangerous patient exception" is a strong limitation to the rule of confidentiality. Of course, while not stipulated, "others" refers to humans. Particularly, in legal and judicial contexts, animals are property rather than persons, and "others" refers only to the latter (Francione 1995).

A second exception to the client-therapist privilege involves laws and professional codes that safeguard children from harm by a client. In all 50 states, therapists are mandated to report knowledge of such threats to the safety of a child. "Harm" here is generally more broadly defined than in the Tarasoff laws. In recent times, the elderly, as another class of more vulnerable victims, have been added as a further exception or limitation to therapist-client confidentiality. Again, while arguably also a vulnerable class of potential victims, animals are not included.

Finally, a limitation on confidence in the client-provider relationship in veterinary medical practice is relevant here. In this context, "client" refers to the human seeking care for his or her companion animal. The American and Canadian Veterinary Medical Associations, the American Animal Hospital Association, and national veterinary associations in the United Kingdom and New Zealand have established policies declaring that veterinarians have responsibilities to protect animal welfare and report suspected animal abuse to relevant authorities. The evolution of these policies coincides with the profession's increasing recognition of the connections between animal abuse and other forms of family violence (Arkow 2015a).

Although current legislation and professional codes governing client-therapist confidentiality do not support or even allow the therapist to break confidence to report animal abuse or a reasonable prospect of animal abuse, these three exceptions provide precedents and openings for such policy innovations. Of course, in most instances therapists are working with clients whose animal abuse is of public record, and the issue here is the obligation or permission to report prospective abuse. Minimally, policy might be developed that, while not mandating reporting animal abuse, protects the therapist from civil and criminal liability for making a report in good faith. This can be argued for the sake of an animal or, as suggested by AVMA policy, for the sake of humans as well, given the established co-occurrence of violent behavior. As animal abuse, at least of companion animals, is widely regarded as socially unacceptable behavior, legal protection for prospective targets of animal abuse should garner significant public support.

However, there is, currently, no clear legal or profession-based protection for therapists who report prospective animal abuse, and, as discussed, the self-selection of therapists who are particularly sensitive to the well-being of animals produces a strong pull toward taking action to protect animals. Absent more progressive policy, we offer the following suggestions.

As in all counseling, the therapist should spell out the limits of confidentiality at the beginning of treatment. This includes specifying what information the therapist may be obligated to present to other agencies such as the courts and the therapist's duty to warn regarding danger to self or other humans. The issue of reporting prospective animal abuse should be discussed with the client and could issue in a signed agreement stipulating the therapist's intention to report such, although it is doubtful that the agreement would be binding either in legal or professional ethics contexts. Clearly, we are in an area here where there is as yet no satisfactory policy and therapists must make their own decisions.

Honesty

In the section on goals and the "true intentions" exercise, we discussed the issue of client (and therapist) honesty largely in the context of the client's understandable reluctance to provide an accurate or full account of his or her treatment of animals. However, in addition to this situationally based pull toward concealment or distortion, many adults who abuse animals, like perpetrators of other forms of abuse, are more generally disposed to dishonesty. They are often individuals who "act out" or externalize their difficulties in living rather than internalize problems and self-blame. To maintain a posture of "I am OK, others are not," requires significant distortion and deceit to the point where it becomes the habitual and preferred form of transaction with others. The following exercise addresses this issue and is intended to be used in initial sessions as part of the framing of the therapy.

Exercise: No Free Rides

The concept of the free ride is simple: those who deceive others think they are getting away with something. The point of this exercise is that there is always a price for deception; it undermines relationships and promotes self-serving behavior that is maladaptive. The metaphor of "no free rides" establishes that misrepresentations have consequences—that they create a web in which someone is caught and may be hurt.

The exercise requires that the therapist be assertive in questioning the client about statements which are, or appear to be, deceptive, explaining to the client that learning to identify and avoid taking free rides is essential to the success of the therapy. The therapist will want the client to learn that deception undermines the necessary trust between therapist and client and also undermines trust in other relationships.

Once the therapist has explained this concept, he or she can confront subsequent client deceptions by saying, "No free rides" or "It sounds like you are trying to take a free ride here." With some clients, the therapist may need to intervene often with statements such as, "Let's think about what you are saying. There are no free rides here." The therapist can explain to the client that this deception is not free—some creature in the living environment is paying for it and so is the client, since deception contributes to his or her alienation from others.

This kind of assertiveness is more difficult for therapists than one might expect. Most of us are taught that it is rude to question people who appear to be sincere. Some clients expect the therapist to be easily deceived. Therapists-in-training are usually taught the value of accepting clients unconditionally. Therapists, however, who accept client accounts at face value will severely limit their understanding of client dynamics and will miss the opportunity to have effective intervention with a substantial number of clients. Therapists who appropriately confront client deception, on the other hand, often find that their clients feel affirmed because someone cared enough to probe into their problems and to understand the emotional pain behind their deception. If the therapist is skilled, *No Free Rides* will come across as playful encouragement rather than accusation. *No Free Rides* is a creative way to confront clients and also allows the client to internalize the principle. It does require delicacy for the therapist is questioning the client as to whether or not he or she is lying. The therapist must be able to state unpleasant realities in a matter-of-fact manner without turning the confrontation into a condemnation of the client's morals.

Several options are available to help a therapist discover whether a client is being deceptive. First, the therapist can use information gained in sessions to clarify inconsistencies. Second, in some agencies the therapist can use information from a client's records to point out where the client is shading the truth. Third, the therapist can use information from referral sources (such as judges, probation officers, or prosecutors) to confront a client's deception.

The exercise depends on some measure of trust and at the same time provides an opportunity to further establish trust. As trust builds, the client should be able to internalize the experience and monitor his or her inclination to take a free ride.

Clinical Case
See Sect. 4.1 for a brief description of Abby. After checking the court report, the therapist confronts Abby with her deception about her boyfriend's dog. As we will discuss immediately below, the deception is part of the story clients often tell to justify their abusive behavior. "Abby, I think you are not being straight with me here. According to the court, your boyfriend denies that his dog bit you and you were unable to show any evidence of the bite at the trial." After she replies sticking to her story, the therapist states, "I have to tell you, there are no free rides with deception. You are paying a high price for this— not only for yourself but for your relationship with Allen. You have said you want him to forgive you, but how can he trust you if he feels you lied to him?" With further discussion, Abby reveals that the dog only growled at her and that she had always been afraid of dogs. The therapist

suggests that she talk to Allen about her fears and then states, "So let's have a working agreement that when I believe you are not telling the truth, I will call you on it, and you can do the same with me."

> For another example of the use of this exercise, see Demonstration DVD, Clinical Exercises submenu, Clinical Exercise #2. See Sect. 4.1 for a brief description of this client—"John."

Homework Assignment
Ask the client to keep a written record of conversations he or she has had with friends and family members throughout the week in which he or she tried to take a "free ride." Go over the record and help the client clarify his or her motivations for deception and speculate on the cost to the person who was deceived, the client, and the relationship.

3.2   Establishing Accountability

Failure of clients to be accountable or accept responsibility for their actions and feelings is often one component of the larger issue of resistance to therapy and the willingness or ability to change. Some form of resistance is part of many, if not most, clients' initial and often enduring self-presentation. Dealing with it is a defining feature of the major therapy approaches. The client-centered therapist joins the client, exploring and reflecting on the circumstance and self-presentation—"what are your feelings about being here?" The psychodynamic therapist encourages associations to the current circumstance—"so you experienced this feeling of undeserved blame when you were a child." The cognitive-behaviorist identifies and clarifies with the client the beliefs and behaviors that led to and maintain resistance—"so you assume that you live in a just world."

As is frequently the case with perpetrators of domestic violence (Rosenbaum and Maiuro 1989), adults who abuse animals frequently refuse to accept responsibility for their actions. A common presenting position is "I have no idea what I am doing here. This is ridiculous." Again, often the position is in the context of court proceedings in which the client is defending against charges of animal abuse. As we will discuss, when presented in that limited context in an otherwise generally compliant client, it is not a serious obstacle to the therapy. However, in clients where it is a more general stance, it is a major deterrent to any constructive movement in the therapy. For this reason, it should be addressed in the treatment as early as possible. Given the goal of eliminating the behavior of animal abuse at some point in the therapy, this population of clients must examine the abusive nature of their actions and see the abuse as something that they can control.

Often a major part of a client's initial self-presentation, denial of accountability frequently takes the form of a justificatory story: "I am just here because the judge told me I had to be here"; "it was just an animal"; "it was me or him"; "if you can shoot a deer, you can kick a dog." These rationalizing stories are a serious block to developing a working relationship. Yet without some acceptance of responsibility and admission of some need to change, reduction in the target behavior, animal abuse, is unlikely to occur. The therapeutic catch-22 is that for a major segment of this population, focusing on the presenting story is counterproductive for it can help the client rehearse, amplify, and refine it, which, in turn, results in further commitment to and identification with the story.

In our experience, it is useful to assess for and distinguish between three levels of resistance. In the "compliant client," resistance is minimal and the typical position is: "look, the judge told me to come here, I am here, I won't fight you, you do your job and I'll do mine." The "resistant client" insists that he or she "…didn't do anything wrong" or that the judge got it all wrong." The system messed up, at least in this instance. For the "defensive client," the externalized position shared by the resistant client is rigidly held and part of a more generally held position—it is always the system's, the other person's, or the animal's fault or problem.

3.2.1 The Compliant Client

Compliance is not a common self-presentation in this population. As the target behavior of animal abuse is often a form of acting out, most clients externalize and/ or have impulse control problems. The occasional compliant client is more internalized. Anxiety, depression, frustration, and loss are immediately felt or at least readily available. Here are two examples (for additional case material on these two clients, see Sect. 4.1, "Ted" and "Aaron"):

> Ted, a 38-year-old computer programmer, lives alone. Although he is very competent at his work, he has few social skills and no intimate friends. His conviction for animal cruelty came from poisoning a number of feral cats, whom he claimed kept him up at night.
> In the initial assessment, the therapist determined that Ted was suffering from depression and advised him to be evaluated for medication. He complied and was placed on a combination of two antidepressant drugs. Within 2 weeks he reported feeling some mild improvement, especially in his ability to sleep. The therapist picked up on this prior sleeping difficulty and his poisoning of the cats and began to explore a possible relationship.
> The therapist observed that Ted had a long history of difficulty with sleeping, which was one symptom of his depression. She wondered whether the cats had really kept him up at night or if he had some other motivation for killing them.
> Ted, at first, wanted to avoid this area of exploration. But with patience and persistence, the therapist was able to engage Ted in thinking about this connection. She had him think in great detail about his feelings before, during, and after the cats' deaths. In revisiting that time, Ted responded: "I guess I was feeling at rock bottom. It was 3 o'clock in the morning and I hadn't slept well for days. And those cats were making that hollering noise—it is spooky. After I decided to poison them I guess I felt a kind of 'rush.' At least I was doing something about the problem. It's weird, but I felt energized in a way."
> He went on to say that he didn't want to beat up on himself for killing the feral cats, claiming "they probably didn't have long to live anyway." Then he continued, stating, "But I don't think I would do that again. Now I have found some relief with the medication."

Aaron was ordered by the courts to undergo counseling when he was convicted of animal cruelty. He beat his own dog, Lady, with a hammer, nearly killing her, when she ran after a squirrel in the park instead of coming to him when he called her.

In treatment Aaron acknowledged that the reason he became so furious with Lady was that she misbehaved in front of a group of his friends. In the first two weeks of treatment, exploration revealed that Aaron had bragged to his friends about how he had trained her.

The therapist remarked that Aaron's self-esteem and sense of self-worth seemed to be closely tied to how well Lady obeyed him, especially when others were looking. He acknowledged that this was the case. This led to a conversation about Aaron's sense that he had to prove himself in order to gain respect. During this conversation, Aaron was unable to see that his deeply felt belief that he had to gain others' respect was a perception and not necessarily a fact of life. He did, however, begin to understand that Lady did not behave in a way to cause him injury, saying: "I still get mad when I think of her 'dissing' me that way, but I guess she probably didn't mean to do it. I mean she didn't mean no disrespect…I know that now, I guess."

For these two clients, the first depressed and withdrawn, and the second whose overidentification with his dog leaves him vulnerable to narcissistic injury, the issues described above under framing the therapy—setting goals, discussing the limits of confidentiality, and the importance of client and therapist being honest— may be sufficient conditions to reduce resistance so that work on the target behavior of animal abuse can proceed.

But denial of accountability in an otherwise compliant client can be present that is not directly motivated by resistance to the therapy. Many clients have subculturally grounded views of animals that condone or even support behaviors toward them that are inconsistent with mainstream cultural norms and with the law. Although sometimes these views are screens for underlying psychological issues, often they are not. Even if the former, the therapist may need to deal with the subcultural issues first to reveal the underlying issues.

In many subcultures (and some mainstream cultures), animals are not considered members of the moral community. Because they do not count as moral beings, humans have no obligations in regard to them and being accountable to them makes no sense. Rather than appropriate objects of moral consideration, they can be treated as property, commodities, instruments, or resources for our use. For those interested in the philosophical literature on the ethics of our treatment of animals, see Regan on rights theory (1983), Singer's utilitarianism (1975), Donovan and Adams' feminist theory (1996), Rowland's contractarianism (1998), Midgley's communitarianism (1983), and Nussbaum's capability theory (2011).

We suggest four ways to deal with subcultural views that support or justify animal abuse by defining animals as beings in regard to whom being accountable makes no sense and is therefore unnecessary:

1. *Offer the client education about the nature of animals.* By staying with the rudiments of animal behavior and skirting the philosophical or ethical issues, the therapist can sometimes avoid a tug-of-war over conflicting mainstream cultural and subcultural views. A client can be given written or video material that deals with the species of animal that he or she abused. As indicated in the introduction,

most of the clients presenting with animal abuse have abused *companion* animals. Material is available from the major national animal protection organizations (e.g., the Humane Society of the United States and the American Society for the Prevention of Cruelty to Animals) or from local humane societies that provide descriptions of the interests, needs, and capabilities of a particular species and of the components of responsible care. Although educational material can complement other interventions that deal with establishing accountability, for compliant clients this may be an adequate intervention.

2. *Explore the client's current or past relationships with animals or relationships observed by the client.* This may reveal aspects of a human-animal relationship that belie his or her subcultural views. A client may respect and treat responsibly individuals of one species but not those of the species abused, or a relative or friend may have treated an animal in ways that even the client finds objectionable. For an exercise involving this latter, see the "Intergenerational Accountability" exercise (p. 47). Examination of these can provide leverage for a soft challenge to the subcultural views that otherwise sustain or allow animal abuse.

3. *Have the client role-play an animal.* Some clients may not be comfortable with or capable of adopting another being's point of view, and this option may need to be delayed until the client is taught the skill of empathizing. See the empathy exercises below. If known, select an animal of a species with whom the client has some history of a positive relationship. For this group of clients, it is not recommended to choose an animal from the species that the client has abused. Again, a successful role-play may produce aspects of an animal—his or her needs or interests—that are inconsistent with and therefore provide a challenge to the client's views.

4. *Explore the subcultural views via values clarification.* Identify values implicit in the subcultural views that, reframed, do not support the animal abuse. For example, a client that hunts animals may be helped to reflect on his or her own abusive behavior as inconsistent with the rules of good sportsmanship that are part of hunting codes.

3.2.2 The Resistant Client

As indicated, we find it useful to distinguish between the resistant client whose denial of accountability is more situational (a reaction to the court mandate) and a client for whom the resistance is a personality trait. Although usually presenting with a story that justifies the abuse without owning it, the former's story is not part of an entrenched defensive posture. It is, however, often accompanied by a strong sense of entitlement. "I can treat animals any way I choose." Furthering the resistance against accepting any responsibility is the sense also that "I am also entitled not to be questioned about it."

According to their theoretical bent, therapists can use particular concepts to break through the story and the entitlement and to establish accountability. However, each in its own way includes risk by providing the client with an occasion to rehearse and reinforce the justificatory story. For examples, the cognitive-behaviorist's notions of overgeneralization and minimization risk losing the emotional component of the behavior; the psychodynamically oriented therapist's denial, rationalization, and projection risk blaming the past; and the client-centered therapist's acceptance and reflection risk validating the abuse. The following exercise is intended to make an end run around the resistance, the sense of entitlement, and unproductive and tension-producing exchanges over the veracity of the client's story.

Exercise: Becoming the Victim
This exercise can be used early in the therapy, as early as the first session, and before the client has staked out a strong denial of accountability and before other patterns of resistance have become a significant part of the therapist-client interaction. The exercise is designed to help the client acknowledge the suffering of the animals and his or her role as the perpetrator of that suffering.

Disrupting the general flow of the conversation, the therapist issues a mild challenge to the client:

> We'll come back to your feelings about what brings you here, but, first, would you be willing to try something with me? We have found that, for clients like you, it is helpful to think of the animal that you abused (or neglected) by imagining yourself as that animal: by putting yourself in that animal's place. What would it be like? What would you, as that animal, be thinking or feeling?

The resistant client may refuse to take this request seriously or deny that he or she ever abused an animal. For most resistant clients, these responses can be readily dealt with—"you've nothing to lose by trying it." Once engaged in the role-play, it is important for the therapist to help the client stay in role by asking the client to keep his or her account in the first person or providing further inquiry about the experience of the animal.

As the purpose of the exercise is to establish accountability, neither the genuine use of empathy by the client nor the veracity of the attempt to describe the experience of the animal is critical. As we will describe in the section on teaching empathy, many people who have difficulty taking up a genuinely empathic posture have learned to "talk the talk" of empathy. In that they present a socially acceptable description, they sound like they are being empathic but are not actually empathizing. Although empathy is an important interpersonal skill, appropriate description not based on empathy can be adequate in many contexts, including the present therapy. In any case, at this point in the therapy what is critical is that through the role-play the client accepts the fact of the suffering and that this acknowledgment serves to undercut the denial of accountability.

Homework Assignment
Provide the client with material, preferably a DVD that portrays an abused animal. Ask the client to write a description of 200 or more words from that animal's perspective, focusing on the animal's pain and suffering.

For an example of the use of this exercise with a mildly resistant client, see Demonstration DVD, Clinical Exercises submenu, Clinical Exercise #1. See Sect. 4.1 for a brief description of this client—"Roy." Note how the therapist deals with the client's initial resistance and helps to keep him in role.

3.2.3   The Defensive Client

Although, as discussed, there are many paths to animal abuse, a common one stems from a rigid defensive posture that can be a serious block to establishing accountability and, more generally, to forming a working therapeutic relationship. These clients are unlikely to work with the therapist by "becoming the victim." While the resistant client's denial of accountability is situational, the defensive client's is part of his or her general personality.

See Demonstration DVD, Clinical Exercises submenu, Clinical Exercise #2 for an initial session with a defensive client. Note how the rigidity of his defensive posture presented a serious challenge to the therapist that degenerated into a battle of wills and likely strengthened the presenting justificatory story. As discussed earlier, it also elicited a countertransference reaction that further detracted from the effectiveness of the intervention.

We describe three approaches to dealing with this subpopulation of defensive clients:

1. *Backdoor approach.* In cases where the denial of accountability is in the context of a defensive posture that includes serious cognitive distortion, it may be advisable to delay the task of establishing accountability to a later phase of the therapy. The therapist buys some time in which to effect some form of working relation, although one not yet built on the shared goal of ending the behavior of animal abuse. This can be done by exploring areas at some distance from the presenting problem and using the therapist's preferred style. For example, in the case of "John" who exercised his dog by chaining him to the back of his moving car (Appendix A 4.1), the therapist could explore John's work situation, perhaps discovering that his work was generally frustrating. Not only did he feel no support from his spouse, he also felt burdened with chores and responsibilities at home that, in his view, his spouse should have been carrying out. This might lead to an exploration of the day in which the incident with the dog occurred, when his wife was out and the kids' toys were blocking the entrance to the house and, of course, no one had walked the dog. The therapist, then, might use these "extenuating" circumstances to help the client own his primary responsibility for the abuse of his dog.
2. *Establish accountability in others.* Unlike the direct challenge of *Becoming the Victim* and like the backdoor approach, the following exercise uses indirection to establish accountability.

Exercise: Intergenerational Accountability

This exercise gets at accountability indirectly by helping the client to acknowledge its presence or absence in another member of his family. To provide material, the therapist inquires about the client's family history, keying on human-animal relationships found in the family history. Some of this material will already be available through the assessment. "Were there any pets in your family when you were growing up? Did your grandparents have any? Who took care of them? How were they disciplined?"

"So your Uncle Henry lived up in Maine and he had a dog that he kept outside through the long winter and the dog was on a chain that was about 12 ft long." Once having identified and explored such a relationship, the critical move is for the therapist to reframe any family member's neglectful or abusive treatment of an animal as irresponsible, wrong, or bad. This move may be unfamiliar or uncomfortable for some therapists as it is clearly distinguished from and may be incompatible with helping the client to understand his own feelings and motivations and those of others through empathy and exploration. Rather than encouraging and reinforcing an empathic response in the client to Uncle Henry, "That must have been tough for Uncle Henry as he really did not have time to deal with the dog"; the therapist is asking, "Is there a way that Uncle Henry might have dealt with the dog in a different—a more responsible and caring—way?" The client may respond by defending his uncle's actions, falling back, at least implicitly, on the subcultural practices to which the client was exposed as a child. "That's how people live with dogs in Maine: They leave them outside, they have thick coats, they do fine." The therapist would then introduce one of the four interventions related to subcultural issues described early under the heading, the compliant client.

Reframing the behavior as wrong is consistent with Jory's Intimate Justice approach which, as indicated, was the primary theoretical basis for the first edition and which we have de-emphasized in this second edition. Still, particularly in the present context, it is helpful for the therapist to introduce terms like "responsibility," "accountability," and "fairness." "Do you think the way that Uncle Henry treated his dog was necessary or fair?" Even a qualified client agreement to this query can be built on to establish accountability as an issue in people's treatment of animals and, eventually, his own treatment of animals.

Homework Assignment

Ask the client to construct a genogram, a diagram of present and past family members that includes companion animals. If helpful, the therapist can share with the client the finding that 99 % of American families consider household animals as family members or close companions (American Veterinary Medical Association 2012). For sample genograms, see McGoldrick and Gerson (1985). Once the genogram is completed, ask the client to describe all the human-animal relationships. The therapist can work with the client to generate descriptive categories and make sure that those related to accountability are included: caring, responsibility, and fairness.

3. *Listening for ambivalence.* Motivational interviewing (MI) is a recent innovation in counseling technique which its developers define as "a client-centered, directive method for enhancing intrinsic motivation to change by exploring and resolving ambivalence" about change (Miller and Rollnick 2002, p. 25). Csillik describes two major components of MI, the relational and the technical (2013, p. 351). The relational reflects the fact that the approach is a development of Rogerian therapy and emphasizes client-centered and nondirective therapist postures such as empathy, affirmation, and reflection. Some of these are consistent with what we have described in the "Joining" subsection of the "Initial Phase of Therapy."

However, as discussed, we have found more directive approaches generally more effective with adults who abuse animals. Miller and Rollnick do describe the technical component, the second component and the one that primarily concerns us here, as involving both nondirective and directive interventions (p. 97).

The technical component refers to ways of eliciting and maintaining "change talk" (Csillik 2013, p. 351). Like denial of accountability, the absence of change talk is a form of resistance to the therapy (Miller and Rollnick, p. 46) and can be a block to progress in the therapy. The therapist works to elicit change talk by identifying the client's ambivalence about making changes in his or her behavior and/or attitudes. Arguably, at some level people have mixed feelings about most of the ways they act and view themselves and others. By listening for explicit or implicit indications of this ambivalence toward the target behavior, the therapist then can help the client to explore both poles of the ambivalence.

With regard to establishing accountability, the identification of ambivalence about taking responsibility for the abuse of an animal is a significant first step. Through the exploration and confirmation of the positive pole ("…that part of you that does feel some responsibility"), the therapist helps the client to accept responsibility for the target behavior.

Clinical Case

The following example is an elaboration of the role-play with John (Sect. 4.1: "John") to illustrate the identification and exploration of ambivalence about accountability:

John: *I really don't think what I did was wrong and anyway it's nobody business but mine. But, obviously, some people don't agree with me or I wouldn't have to be here talking to you – and I have to pay for it!*

Therapist: *And I appreciate that you came and we can talk more about your feelings about being here. Is there anybody else besides the court and the counseling that doesn't agree with you?*

John: *Well, my wife and kids really miss the dog and blame me for what happened even though, like I said, the dog needed exercise and they weren't doing it.*

Therapist: *So, how are you dealing with their feelings?*

John: *Mostly I told my wife that I was pissed that it was her that wanted the dog for the kids and she doesn't walk the dog – and, of course, the kids don't. But I said I would get another dog for the kids.*

Therapist: *So part of you does regret what happened.*

John: *Well, I am sorry the dog died because he couldn't hack it because he was out of shape from not exercising.*

Therapist: *It sounds like you have mixed feelings about what happened to the dog. I understand you have feelings about your wife not taking care of the dog and feel she is partly responsible for what happened, but what would it be like if you also accepted at least some responsibility?*

John: *Like I said I didn't do anything wrong.*

Therapist: *But you did think about the dog's condition – that he was out of shape. I wonder if you thought through whether it was a good idea to exercise him that way?*

John: *Look, I work all day and then have to take care of the dog. I don't have time to…*

Therapist: *Taking care of a dog is a bit like being a parent or advising people about whether to take out a loan. Would you make decisions about your kids or your loan applicants without thinking it through?*

John: *So you're saying I don't have good judgment – but it's only a dog.*

Therapist: *You do feel sorry the dog died. But, partly because you were angry at your wife for not carrying her load, you didn't think through how to deal with the dog. I understand that for the most part you do not feel responsible. I wonder if you can speak from that part of you that* does *feels some responsibility for what happened.*

Conclusion

We have given considerable attention to establishing accountability for two reasons: (1) Without it, reaching the goal of ending animal abuse is unlikely, and (2) for this population, denial of responsibility is a common way of dealing with problems. While we have focused on its relation to the target behavior of ending animal abuse, taking responsibility for or owning his or her feelings also is a general posture that the client can learn through the therapy.

3.3   Interpersonal Skills: Empathy

In the first subsection on intervention strategies, we showed how therapists can form a working relationship with clients and reach agreement on mutually acceptable goals. In the second, we dealt with ways of circumventing resistance to the therapy, focusing on the denial of accountability. The next step is for the client to learn alternative ways of dealing with animals through the acquisition of interpersonal skills. The justification for the emphasis on interpersonal relationships is that it provides a powerful framework for understanding and ending animal abuse. Much therapy is an attempt to help clients form and maintain positive relationships. What we are adding here is the importance of such in our dealings with nonhuman animals. As indicated in the review of the literature on human-animal relationships, most caretakers of companion animals consider them as members of the family. For better or for worse, they play complex roles in the family system.

We can think of the therapy as an attempt to help clients move from negative to positive relationships with animals. Since how people treat other humans and animals is correlated and since similar skills are applicable to both, the effort includes the general development of interpersonal skills. With respect to both their human and animal relationships, the therapist seeks movement from those that are exploitative, controlling, disempowering, and debasing to those that are respectful, empowering, and mutually beneficial. As means to these ends, we discuss ways to increase clients' ability to form and maintain accommodating, reciprocal, and nurturing relationships. We begin with empathy as, arguably, it is an important foundation for these other skills.

3.3.1   Introduction

Empathy is an important and, really, wondrous phenomenon that allows people to have access to and share the experience of other individuals. Although, as we will describe, it has a strong constitutional basis, it is also a skill that can be learned. Ascione (1992) showed that a modest humane education curriculum increases the level of children's empathy and carries over to increased empathy to humans. In the other direction, research has found that higher scores on a measure of empathy toward other humans significantly predict positive attitudes toward animals and disapproval of animal mistreatment (Erlanger and Tsytsarev 2012).

Decastro et al. (2010) refer to empathy as an "umbrella term" that encompasses emotional contagion, perspective-taking, and sympathy. These three empathic processes are complexly related and often are concurrently experienced. However, for the purposes of this handbook, we distinguish them as follows: Emotional contagion is the immediate experience of the distress, anxiety, or joy of another individual. It is evident in infants who "catch" their mother's anxiety. Perspective-taking refers to experiencing the world from another individual's point of view. While never fully achieved, perspective-taking provides a more articulated understanding of a person's situation and needs than does the global emotional sharing of emotional contagion. Sympathy is an emotional response that is reactive to but is not imitative of another individual's feelings. As it is synonymous with compassion and this latter term is more commonly used in the relevant research literature, we will use the terms interchangeably in what follows. As indicated by the following statement, compassion does not necessarily imply a direct sharing of or experiencing another individual's emotional state or situation—"It is hard for me to imagine the pain you are going through, but I feel bad for you." However, emotional contagion and perspective-taking often lead to compassion, a defining feature of which is motivation to alleviate another individual's negative state.

Recent research has established a neurological basis for empathy. Mirror neurons are brain cells that are activated both when a person has a particular feeling or behaves in a particular way and when he or she perceives someone else having the same feeling or performing the same action (Rizzolatti et al. 1996; Di Pellegrino et al. 1992). When a person stubs his toe, the same part of an observer's sensory-motor cortex is stimulated as in the individual observed. The evolution of this special class of neurons hardwires us to imitate, to learn by observing, and to cooperate with and share in the feelings of others. It makes us into social animals. Of course, we are not the only social animals, and, in fact, mirror neurons were first discovered in monkeys in a laboratory setting, regrettably, in the context of highly invasive research (Rizzolatti et al. 2006).

Mirror neurons are the direct physiological basis for emotional contagion. Our apprehension of the emotions of others, particularly the more basic feelings, such as anger, sadness, fear, and joy (DeCastro et al. 2010), involves automatic mechanisms that occur with no effortful processing or cognitive perspective-taking. Through the activation of mirror neurons, an observer immediately experiences feelings comparable to those of the observed individual. The fact that through evolution other animals also developed mirror neurons has important implications for human-animal relationships as it suggests that at least some of our feelings for and attachments to other animals may be reciprocal as well as evolutionarily advantageous. With respect to abusive relationships, an abused animal immediately senses the presumably negative feelings of the human abuser. This may contribute to the perpetuation of violent interactions. It has been found that 21.1 % of animals that caused human fatalities due to dog bites had been abused (Patronek et al. 2013).

The presence of mirror neurons is likely a prerequisite for perspective-taking and at least an important facilitator of sympathy, both of which require more sophisticated cognitive processing.

Empathic responses, then, are an important basis for facilitating the formation of and maintenance of relationships, both human and animal. It also provides an anchoring for the moral judgments made in those relationships (Shapiro et al. 2014, pp. 25, 37). In the context of animal abuse committed as part of domestic violence, dominance and control often substitute for empathy. While the literature clearly demonstrates that empathy correlates with prosocial behavior (Eisenberg and Miller 1987), empathy may also be used as an instrument of control. Through empathy, the perpetrator of domestic violence may understand the closeness of a partner's attachment to a particular companion animal and use that knowledge for dominance and control. As we will describe, particularly in the target populations of AniCare, this makes it critical that the therapist also teach the client compassion as it includes taking prosocial action.

As with many other skills, particularly those involving emotions, there is considerable individual variation in these empathic skills, based on differences in both constitution and socialization. For this reason, therapists should devote special attention to their assessment.

3.3.2   Assessment of Empathy

Through an informal assessment in the course of the initial sessions and a developmental history keying on relationships to humans and animals, the therapist can determine the client's present level of empathic skill. A more formal assessment can be made through administration of an empathy scale (Bryant 1982; Davis 1983). The Bryant scale includes two items specific to empathizing with an animal (Bryant, items 11 and 16).

The following graded list provides a rough guide to the client's current level of empathic skill, beginning with the least developed:

1. The client has limited capacity and vocabulary to express his own feelings.
2. The client does not demonstrate empathic behavior even following the therapist's prompt—"Imagine what it might have been like to be that individual…."
3. The client does not spontaneously demonstrate empathic behavior but can in response to a simple prompt.
4. The client does not currently demonstrate empathic behavior even in response to a simple prompt, but his history suggests that he at one time had that capacity.
5. The client demonstrates empathic behavior to people but not animals.
6. The client demonstrates empathic behavior to some individual animals or individuals of some species but not others (e.g., dogs but not cats).

As suggested, the therapist should distinguish the three components of empathy discussed earlier and various combinations and permutations. A client may demonstrate emotional contagion but not perspective-taking such that he is limited to basic and relatively generalized emotional responses—"that guy (dog) is angry—I can just feel it" and he may or may not sympathize ("I sure am glad I am not him"). Another client can take a perspective on another's experience, but it is largely a cognitive understanding rather than an emotional appreciation of the individual's situation and may or may not include sympathizing.

Another consideration is assessing the possibility that the client is faking it. Particularly in a subpopulation that often includes psychopathic and related self-presentations, some individuals will talk like they are empathizing, but their experience of the other individual is limited to inference based on a reading of the situation—"If I was in that situation, I would feel…." Distinguishing mouthing the feelings from really feeling what the other felt requires careful observation by the therapist. As we will discuss, for some clients this pseudo-empathy may be the best adjustment.

As suggested in items #5 and #6 above, people learn through socialization those categories in their environment that are considered appropriate objects of empathy. Given the hardwired tendency to empathize, children often empathize with inanimate objects—e.g., the toast that jumped out of the toaster because it was burning. Regarding empathy with animals, they must learn nonobvious and complex distinctions—the animals on their plate and those that are members of the family; the animals that are reduced to pests and those that are made human-like (the mouse in the trap and Mickey Mouse, respectively; Shapiro 1990). Part of the assessment, then, is to identify the client's categories of appropriate objects of empathy and to understand their source, whether it be family of origin, broader subculture, or individual dynamics. This will suggest the level of intervention necessary to broaden the client's use of empathy and to make it consistent with socially acceptable behavior toward animals.

Finally, it is important to assess the client's current emotional reaction to the actual presence of animals as this will affect whether and when to include a live animal as a vehicle for teaching empathy as well as other interpersonal skills. Reactions may range from callous and indifferent to traumatized and guilty (Gupta 2008). The reactions may be limited to individuals of a particular species or they may be general. The therapist can evaluate client reactions by varying the degree of direct presence of an animal, beginning with the most indirect, such as a story about an animal, to the actual presence of an animal in the session. We return to this issue in the discussion of animal-assisted therapy and activities below.

3.3.3 Intervention

We organize interventions for the development of empathic skills in terms of the three processes discussed—emotional contagion, perspective-taking, and compassion.

3.3.4 Emotional Contagion: *How Do You Think He Felt?*

Although in its developed form it is a highly sophisticated cognitive ability, in its precursor form empathy is closer to a reflexive response. People are immediately aware of another individual's emotion even before they put it into words. The sense of the feelings of another individual, whether human or animal, can be immediately apprehended. From an early age, a child who sees someone being kicked has an immediately given sense of pain. This unlearned response is so general that it even can be elicited with the cartoon-like presentation of geometric figures "interacting" (Piaget 1926).

Through the arousal of the hardwired system of mirror neurons, even the most defended client will spontaneously experience a feeling similar to that of another individual involved in an obviously emotional situation. The therapist can attempt to elicit an empathic client response to any material, whether presented by the client or introduced by the therapist—such as in response to a story or picture involving an animal. However, in individuals with poor empathic skills (#1 and #2 above), that feeling may be provided with little elaboration and may be limited to the basic emotions that are associated with emotional contagion.

Some clients have limited awareness both of the feelings of others and of their own feelings. While it is possible that some clients may be so other-directed that they can empathize with others but are not in touch with their own feelings, the two deficits generally occur together. In some people, the failure of awareness even may extend to basic emotions such as anger—e.g., the client with clenched fists who denies he is angry.

In addition to a deficit in awareness, some clients have impoverished vocabularies of feelings that may be confined to those of a young child (mad, sad, bad, and glad). Therapists can provide such clients with exercises and materials that first focus on identifying and naming feelings about self. See the AniCare Child Handbook (Shapiro et al. 2014, pp. 25–30) for material that could be adapted for adults. The following sequence is suggested:

1. Associate the basic emotions with appropriate situations involving the client's emotional reaction.
2. Associate more nuanced feelings (frustrated, envious, rejected, denigrated, etc.) with appropriate situations.
3. For the latter, teach vocabulary consistent with the client's cognitive ability.

The same sequence can then be followed with respect to empathic responses, using the prompt: How do you think he felt?

Once the client has a level of skill consistent with his cognitive ability, the therapist can provide material that features an abusive situation. For discussion of whether to start with human/human or human/animal abuse, see below. It is important to help the client to empathize with both the victim and the perpetrator: How do you think the person kicked felt? How do you think the person doing the kicking felt?

If the client has a history of witnessing abuse, whether human or animal, a further variant is to explore material in which there is a third party observing the abuse: How do you think that child felt watching his father kick their dog? Witnessing abuse can have either a modeling effect, teaching violence as a way to deal with others, or a traumatic effect (Thompson and Gallone 2006) and should be explored as a possible pathway to the client's abusive behavior.

3.3.5 Perspective-Taking: *Tell Me More About How He Felt and Why Do You Think He Felt That Way?*

The exercises in the previous section may elicit material that includes more nuanced, complex, and situated emotions, indicating that the client already is complementing emotional contagion with perspective-taking. However, when that is not the case and where there is no spontaneous empathic response even following simple prompts, the therapist can work more directly on developing the client skill of perspective-taking. The therapist should assess whether the deficit is a function of clients' limited cognitive ability, their belief that animals are unable to or have very limited ability to experience feelings, or individual dynamics—and intervene accordingly.

At the simplest level, perspective-taking is predominantly perceptual and requires minimal cognitive ability. An individual sees what another individual is seeing with only a minimal understanding of the situation and without yet imagining the accompanying intentions, motivations, and interests. The therapist can ask the client to "see" and describe the other side of an object hidden from his view (the other side of the car or bushes seen from the window) ("Yes, I know you can't see it but what do you imagine the other side looks like?"). Next, the therapist asks the client to "see" an object from another individual's physical perspective. See Piaget's classic demonstration of the emerging perspective-taking ability of the child in the "three mountains task" (Mounoud 1996, pp. 113–114). Once the client is comfortable with that limited perspective-taking, he is then encouraged to elaborate: "Tell me more about what the individual was or is thinking and feeling?" The final steps involve taking the perspective of an animal and, eventually, an abused animal.

If these final steps still produce an impoverished account of the animal's experience, the problem may be the lack of knowledge about animals, and it may be helpful to provide the client with educational material about the target species. Depending on the sophistication of the client, the material might be pamphlets produced by national or local animal protection groups, a natural history, or a popular version of a study in cognitive ethology (Balcombe 2006).

If the client provides an account which, while substantial enough, is clearly biased toward negative and impoverished views of animals, the problem may be either with subcultural view or client projection. As discussed in the section on establishing accountability, the bias is generally in the service of justifying his abuse of the animals. In that section, we described four interventions to circumvent subcultural views that support or justify animal abuse (see Sect. 3.2.1). Similarly, for the client clearly projecting his own issues to justify his abusive behavior, we provided three interventions (see Sect. 3.2.3).

As this is a topic that is uniquely germane to working with this population, we add here a brief overview of client accounts of animals. It is helpful to think about client presentations about animals as predominantly a description of (1) the animal-as-such, (2) the animal-as-constructed (Shapiro 2008, pp. 5–6), and, we add here for this population, (3) the animal-as-projected:

- The animal-as-such is consistent with the natural historical and scientific understanding of the animal, e.g., dogs protect a territory.
- The animal-as-constructed is what we have called "subcultural" construction, e.g., dogs should be kept tied up outside even in the harshest weather.
- The animal-as-projected is based on the psychology of the individual, e.g., my dog is better than your dog.

Whatever its basis, the therapist's first priority is to help the client develop an account that supports nonabusive behavior toward the target animals and, by extension, nonabusive and respectful relationships with other animals and with people.

Accounts based primarily on cultural constructions of an animal vary in emphasizing views that, from that subcultural perspective, are positive or negative (wise owl or filthy pig). For the purposes of promoting nonabusive behavior, the therapist can reinforce positive views, even if they are not strictly accurate scientifically. Socially constructed accounts further vary in featuring attributes that distinguish them from humans or that show their similarity to humans (animals don't feel pain like we do, or, like us, animals are very sensitive to having their feelings hurt). As there is an association between accounts that emphasize similarities between humans and animals and higher levels of empathy and sympathy (Clayton et al. 2009), it is better for our purposes if the subcultural construction "errs" on the side of similarities. However, an exception and a final consideration is that the therapist should not reinforce similarities that are not prosocial (humans and other animals are primarily interested in their own survival). We return to the importance of the client's account in a discussion of narrative-based therapy below.

Regarding accounts largely based on individual projections or, more generally, individual client dynamics, the therapist should explore with clients the reasons for their difficulties in perspective-taking. In the case of male clients, part of the problem may be that empathic responses are inconsistent with their self-concept as a man. These clients may use distancing devices to suppress any empathic feelings (Serpell 1986, p. 151). In some clients, strong feelings make the empathic grasp of other individuals' experience difficult or grossly distorted—e.g., anger, superiority, jealousy, or hatred. Exploration of these can lead to other feelings that highlight similarities between the perpetrator and the animal victim. For example, anger may be in the service of blocking feelings of vulnerability. The therapist can work with the client to identify and explore a situation in which he felt vulnerable or, if that is too threatening, someone he knows who felt vulnerable. Once the client has a sense of what vulnerability feels like, a more constructive and accurate empathic response may be possible in which he appreciates that, like him, the abused animal has a strong sense of vulnerability. A disclaimer: Clients in whom preoccupying and distorting emotions, such as anger and hatred, are entrenched and uncritically part of the client's self-concept may need more intensive therapy.

We have discussed several blocks to the constructive use of empathy as a vehicle for reducing abusive behavior and suggested interventions tailored to each. In some cases, role-play may be a more direct and effective way of teaching empathy. In others, the kinds of work we have just discussed are necessary before the client is willing or able to role-play. "Imagine being that individual; describe what he or she experiencing at that moment; describe the experience from his or her point of view."

The sequencing of situations that the therapist asks the client to role-play is important. The therapist should move progressively from situations that are nonthreatening and accessible for the client to those that are more stressful and remote, culminating in empathizing with the animal the client abused. For clients who are more comfortable with relating to humans, the following sequence of targeted objects of empathy is suggested:

- Human in positive situation
- Human in negative situation
- Animal in a positive situation
- Animal in a negative situation
- Animal who has been abused

For clients who have had a strong positive relationship with an animal and who are anxious with or avoidant of humans, the therapist can adjust the sequence accordingly. See AniCare Child Handbook (Shapiro et al., p. 48) for a discussion of sequencing in the context of juvenile who has abused animals.

As even compliant clients may have difficulty staying with this task, it is important for the therapist to gently but firmly keep the client in role. The therapist can suggest that the client use first-person pronouns when describing the experience of the role-played individual ("please say 'I,' not 'he'"). Through simple inquiries ("what happened then?"), the therapist can help the client provide a concrete and detailed account of the situation and go on to describe more psychological aspects of the role-played individual's experience—motivations and intentions. When necessary, the therapist can model role-playing.

As discussed earlier, the therapist should be wary of ersatz forms of empathy. A client may provide responses based on inferentially reading a situation and/or on an analogy to his own experience, rather than on a genuinely empathic move (a person in that situation would feel…; I have been in a similar situation and felt…; therefore, the animal feels…). Although we have been emphasizing ways to acquire the skill, truly empathically based responses may be beyond the reach of some clients. Inferentially and self-referentially based readings of interpersonal situations may be such clients' best adjustment and may suffice to substitute prosocial behavior for abusive behavior.

3.3.6 Compassion: *How Do You Feel About Him Feeling That Way?*

Compassion (or sympathy), the third component of empathic responses, is "feeling for" an individual and is distinguished from empathy which is "feeling with" an individual. Goetz, Keltner, and Simon-Thomasazarus define compassion as "the feeling that arises in witnessing another's suffering and that motivates a subsequent desire to help" (2010, p. 353). This definition clearly differentiates compassion from perspective-taking, which refers to the experience of sensing another individual's situation and feelings. Unlike either emotional contagion or perspective-taking, compassion includes a motivation to act on behalf of the distressed individual. It is related to altruistically prosocial behavior such as the desire to alleviate another individual's distress (Eisenberg and Strayer 1987). Levin and Arluke (2013) found that subjects have a greater compassionate response (reported "emotional distress") for infants, puppies, and mature dogs than they do for adult humans. Shiota et al. (2006) found that people with a strong trait of compassion, as distinguished from a momentary state, have secure attachment styles.

Goetz, Keltner, and Simon-Thomasazarus state that "…compassion evolved as a distinct affective experience whose primary function is to facilitate cooperation and protection of the weak and those who suffer" (2010, p. 351) and that it is "…a proximal determinant of prosocial behavior" (p. 352) to lessen the suffering or distress of other individuals. One argument for its selective advantage is that compassion-based action "enhances the welfare of vulnerable offspring" (p. 357).

We are focusing here on teaching compassion in our clients. However, it is worth noting that, by comparison to perspective-taking, therapists responding compassionately to clients can more readily retain some emotional distance to their distress or suffering. This has important implications for avoidance of therapist emotional fatigue and burnout.

Compassion can be taught to clients. It can be used as a next step following the achievement of adequate perspective-taking or as a substitute for the limits in that skill often found in this population. Feeling other individuals' pain or distress readily leads to feeling badly for them, but one can feel badly for others without first having empathized with them. This may be sufficient occasion to motivate eliminating abusive behavior.

Conversely, uncaring responses to other individuals' pain or suffering are possible when those individuals are felt to be deserving of pain. As discussed, such views are often part of the justificatory story of clients who refuse to accept accountability for their abusive behavior. To develop a compassionate response and story will require that clients reach some level of valuing animals, accept that animals are capable of suffering, and regret being a perpetrator of their suffering.

One form of compassionate action is based on accommodation, an interpersonal skill in which individuals alter their behavior to meet the needs and to alleviate the suffering of others. Often animal abusers are not adept at accommodating, whether to humans or animals. They have relied on dominance to fulfill their own needs and to control others' behavior. Some associate accommodation with weakness or with an admission of fallibility and insist on acting unilaterally. As a result, they often have not developed the basic interpersonal skills that are requisite to accommodating to others' needs, such as listening, understanding, and respecting others' needs. In the case of animals, this can be accomplished through education, direct observation, and/or empathy. According to their theoretical bent, therapists can address the cognitive distortions or dynamics of maladaptive uses of power- and control-based relationships to obtain psychological gratification before identifying and coaching clients in the requisite skills.

Therapists can help clients give up their need to control by recognizing that accommodation is a two-way street in which their own needs also can be met. There is also the satisfaction in being in a relationship that is more equitable and reciprocal as well as the satisfaction of meeting the needs of others. We discuss the latter below in the exercise on nurturance (Sect. 3.4.2).

An important component of accommodation is the skill of negotiating—of working out the terms of who is doing what for whom. Many clients will assume that negotiation with animals is not possible, as their communication with them is one directional and largely limited to giving commands—laying down the law and enforcing it. Through interactions with an animal in the session or reenacting transactions reported by clients, therapists can sensitize them to the various ways that animals communicate and indicate their preferences and intentions. A good example that may be familiar and easy to imagine for many clients is taking a dog for a walk. Clients can become aware of how dogs communicate when they want to go out, where they want to stop and explore, which path they want to take, and when they want to go home. Therapists can readily show clients how, in effect, walking the dog and, in general, any interaction with other animals can involve negotiations in which each party, in turn, can accommodate to the needs and preferences of the other.

Exercise: Fostering Flexibility
Therapists can introduce this exercise by explaining to clients that learning new skills is a good way to replace older ways of behaving that have not served them well. In addition to meeting the needs formerly met by older styles of relating, these new skills can help them achieve other satisfactions that they may have been lacking in past relationships. This exercise can begin with a discussion of human-human interactions in which accommodation is more readily demonstrated—"it's your turn to decide what we are going to do this weekend," or "how about if I fix the screen-door and you get dinner ready." When clients have some understanding of the process, therapists can ask them to examine human-animal interactions, whether with an animal present in the session or through a remembered or imagined animal.

The therapist then can explore interactions for the possible role of accommodation. Did the clients accommodate to the animal's needs? If not, what prevented them from doing so? What were the clients thinking and feeling? From both the animals' and clients' perspectives, how might the outcome of the interaction been different if they had accommodated? It is important that the therapist walk clients step by step through a number of examples of interactions that involve accommodation until they have learned the skill.

> For an example of the use of this exercise, see Demonstration DVD, Clinical Exercises submenu, Clinical Exercise #5. See Sect. 4.1 for a brief description of this client—"Roy."

Clinical Case
Mark was required to participate in counseling after he was convicted of kicking his girlfriend's cat, Binder, down a flight of stairs. The cat was seriously injured and required extensive veterinary care.

In describing the events around the incident, Mark was able to connect the abuse of Binder with his anger at his girlfriend. They had argued the night before after she returned from a night out with her friends. Mark had insisted that she had "disobeyed" him by going out with her girlfriends without consulting him first. He acknowledged that his abuse of Binder might have been a way to retaliate against his girlfriend. With prompting, he described other incidents in their relationship in which he had felt threatened and responded with anger.

The therapist then explored Mark's view of relationships in general. To the query as to what he thought was the most important ingredient in a successful relationship, Mark responded, "having one person be in charge and the other person listening to that person." The therapist asked Mark if this might not be a self-serving definition, since he would probably assign himself the role of the one "being in charge." Mark tried to evade the question at first, but after a while said that "Yes, I guess it does favor me."

The therapist asked Mark to imagine a way in which he might accommodate to his girlfriend's needs and how he thought that might affect her view of him and his view of himself. Again, Mark tried to deflect the request, but after some gentle persistence on the therapist's part, Mark replied: "Well, she comes home late every Wednesday because that is the way her shift works. I guess I could get the dinner together that night even if I just ordered a pizza in, or something….. and I guess that would make her like me or soften up to me. I don't know how I would feel about myself. I might not like everybody knowing about it…but I guess it would be OK."

The therapist then said, "Let's go a step further here. Now try to imagine how you might accommodate to Binder…and then try to imagine how that would affect the cat, and how she responded to you, and also how you felt about yourself." Mark responded by saying, "What? To a cat?" The therapist had to persistently keep Mark on track, but with the therapists' gentle prodding, Mark offered that perhaps Binder would like it if he brought her home a treat every now and then. Finally, after some exploration of his feelings, Mark admitted that sometimes he enjoyed the cat curling up on the sofa with him and his girlfriend and that it was only fair that he did something for the cat in return.

Homework Assignment 1

If providing an animal in the therapy is not feasible, therapists can help clients arrange for direct experiences with animals (in a shelter, sanctuary, or dog training class where adequate supervision is available) to practice accommodation. These experiences can then be discussed in the therapy and appropriate changes suggested.

Homework Assignment 2

Ask clients to offer restitution for their acts of animal abuse. The form of the restitution will vary. In the case of animals that were killed, it might involve doing something for the abused animals' caretaker, such as writing a letter of apology. If that is not feasible, clients could act in the interest of the species of animals involved in the abuse.

3.3.7 Animal-Assisted Therapy

We have described possible sequencing of the targets of empathy based on two variables—human/animal and positive/negative. Another consideration in the therapy is the choice of "materials" used at different points in the sequence. To supplement the animal-related content spontaneously presented by the client or elicited by therapist inquiry, the therapist can introduce animal-related stories, pictures, and, the real thing—an animal.

As empathic processes involve having access to or sharing the experience of other individuals, the actual presence of the object of empathy is important. Particularly in regard to emotional contagion, the most hardwired of the processes, the immediate presence of the object of empathy delivers the access—when people see a door slam on someone's foot, they also pull back in pain. It follows from this that involving a live animal may be an effective way of teaching empathy. However, as we will describe, introducing the actual presence of an animal may be counter-indicated at least at certain points in the process of developing empathy. Fortunately, most individuals can empathize in the absence of the actual object of empathy when prompted by other materials. People empathize with the actor on the cinema screen and the character in the book or by remembering, imagining, or role-playing an interaction.

The therapist can consider a spectrum of materials varying in the directness or indirectness of the presence of the target such as the following, ordered roughly from the most to the least direct:

• Live animal
• Video or pictures of animals
• Client provided incidents involving animals
• Client provided drawings of animals
• Role-played incidents involving animals
• Stories about animals—actual or fictional

When teaching and then using empathy in the therapy, direct materials have the advantage of immediate presence but the possible drawbacks of eliciting defensive reactions, particularly with resistant and defensive clients. Indirect materials require a more imaginative leap but may be less threatening.

More generally, beyond eliciting empathic responses, the therapist should consider the pros and cons of including an actual animal in the therapy depending on the client, the therapist-client relationship, and the phase of the therapy. This then raises the larger question of the use of animal-assisted therapy (AAT) with clients who have abused animals.

The centrality of the role of the animal in AAT can vary. The term "animal-assisted therapy," as distinguished from "animal-assisted activity," is reserved for contexts in which the animals are "an integral part of the therapeutic process" (Pet Partners, 2010)[1]. In many social situations, the presence of an animal facilitates contact between humans. Capitalizing on these findings, therapists can introduce an animal as a facilitator or icebreaker (Zilcha-Mano 2013, p. 123) in the early phases of therapy or throughout the therapy to provide emotional support for the client or to reduce the intensity of unmediated client-therapist contact. The therapist can explore with clients their feelings about the presence of an animal to determine whether, when, and how to involve a live animal. For example, for some clients in this population of adults who have abused animals, the presence of an animal may be stressful, threatening, or, generally, too emotionally laden. In the early phases of therapy, it may complicate the establishment of accountability—"what a nice dog—of course, I would never do anything to hurt an animal."

A live animal can be involved more intensively to explore relationships, both human-animal and human-human. The therapist can take the present and evolving client-animal relationship as a model for other relationships, much as in psycho-dynamic therapy the client-therapist relationship serves that function. As human-animal relationships are often simpler, less ambivalent, and more predictable than human-human relationships, they make useful models (Zilcha-Mano 2013, p. 120). Comfort with intimacy, degree of closeness, form of attachment, sensitivity to rejection, and separation anxiety all can be examined. The therapist also can use the client-animal relationship as a vehicle to teach interpersonal skills (see Sect. 3.4). In that animals are perceived as "forgiving," practicing client interaction with them is a helpful vehicle for honing these skills (Zilcha-Mano 2013, pp. 129, 132).

Attachment Theory

AAT is in a formative stage of development, and many scholars have noted that validation of its effectiveness is not yet established; nor has research identified what aspects of the presence of an animal in the therapy, if any, are therapeutic (Chur-Hansen et al. 2014; Marino 2012). That notwithstanding, a great deal of anecdotal evidence supports its effectiveness, and attachment theory has been offered as an explanation for its putative effectiveness (Zilcha-Mano 2013, pp. 111–144).

According to attachment theory, individuals develop a model of or template for attachments in early childhood that informs later relationships. If that model features insecure attachment issues, it leads to the formation of dismissing,

---

[1] The former Delta Society (now Pet Partners) defines animal-assisted activities as follows: Animal-assisted activities (AAA) provide opportunities for motivational, educational, recreational, and/or therapeutic benefits to enhance quality of life. AAA are delivered in a variety of environments by specially trained professionals, paraprofessionals, and/or volunteers in association with animals that meet specific criteria (Delta Society 2010).

preoccupied, or fearful relationships. Often using the therapist-client relationship as a vehicle, therapists work with clients to replace that model with a more secure attachment. In their review of the literature on animals and attachment theory, Rockett and Carr suggest "that human-animal relationships might… have enormous therapeutic potential… to 'lubricate' the formation of attachment-like relationships in the therapist-client setting" (2014, p. 429). Zilcha-Mano argues that the use of AAT offers an alternative vehicle for this work as an animal can function as an attachment figure (2013, p. 125) and clients may relate to the animal in a way that replicates their insecure attachment model. This provides therapists the opening to examine that relationship and, as with the therapist-client relationship, to help clients replace it with a more secure attachment that generalizes to human-human relationships. The use of the animal-client relationship can be used to avoid the hostility and conflict inherent in therapists' attempts to facilitate a change in the form of a relationship, that of the therapist-client, of which they are one party (Zilcha-Mano, p. 119). See the discussion of attachment disorder in animal hoarders—Sect. 4.4.

As is the current case with AAT, the etiology of animal abuse and what constitutes its effective intervention are not fully understood. A conservative assumption, based on our experience with many cases, is that, like other forms of violence, many paths lead to animal abuse and that one of these is faulty attachments. In the context of juveniles, we suggested that early difficulties with attachment may be one pathway to animal abuse (Shapiro et al., pp. 23–24, 2014) and that attachment theory is a useful frame for understanding it (pp. 100–106).

What we are adding here is that AAT may be an effective way of dealing with that subpopulation of adult clients whose abuse of animals is a result of faulty attachments. The therapist introduces an animal into the session and facilitates the establishment of a client-animal attachment. If that attachment replicates the client's insecure attachment model, the therapist analyzes it with the client and works toward establishing a more secure attachment. Once this is established, the therapist helps the client to substitute prosocial interpersonal skills for abusive forms of interaction.

Animal Welfare

In the earlier section on "Confidentiality," we discussed the problem of dealing with client threats of or actual harm to animals outside the therapy hour. In addition, the therapist should take precautions to assure the safety and welfare of animals in the therapy session. The therapist should closely monitor the degree and nature of client physical contact with animals present in the therapy. The therapist needs to be aware that animals are sensitive to clients' expressions of negative emotions and may respond with their own distress or with aggression. Although clients' anger and aggression toward and frustration with an animal are part of the therapy process and grist for the therapeutic mill, the welfare of the animal should be the first priority (Arkow 2015b, pp. 67–68). Part of the framing of the therapy should be a limit-setting statement by the therapist that no threat to the well-being and safety of any animals in the session will be allowed.

3.4   Other Interpersonal Skills

One of the purposes of the work on empathy described in the first section on interpersonal skills is to help clients to begin to recognize animals as individuals with their own needs, feelings, interests, and preferences. As indicated, therapists can supplement the practice of empathy skills with materials in animal behavior and ethology. In effect, the therapist is reframing animals as autonomous individuals who have their own ways of experiencing the world and who, based on that experience, interact with other individuals both within and across species. Through these interactions, over time an interpersonal relationship is established the form of which is a result of the actions of both parties. In the present context, clients have formed abusive relationships and, as discussed, often have denied to animals the capability of being in a relationship of any form. The therapist needs to train them in interpersonal skills that are, minimally, nonabusive and, ideally, that result in benefits to both parties.

We have discussed several variables in the teaching of interpersonal skills. Here, we review them in the form of the following schema:

- Subjects of the relationship: human or animal
- Valence of the content: negative or positive
- Presence of animals: direct or indirect

When considering an intervention, therapists should think through the selection of the subjects of the relationship (human-human or human-animal) and the valence (positive or negative) of the content. Although often beginning with material primarily involving humans, most interventions eventually will focus on animals, and therapists need to decide on the directness or indirectness of the presence of animals. Therapists should also decide on the most effective presentation sequence of the three variables.

3.4.1   Respect

It follows from the discussion of treating animals as individuals that an important interpersonal skill is respect—how to form and maintain respectful relationships. As with empathy, the skill of relating respectfully can be acquired and/or solidified through the process of acquiring some of the other skills described below. However, arguably, for some skills, learning to interact respectfully with animals is a prerequisite for their acquisition. Without it, there is little incentive to be accommodating or nurturing or caring. With it, the therapist can more effectively work with the client to replace negative, disrespectful, forms of interaction (controlling, dominating, exploiting, and disempowering)—with positive and respectful forms.

Therapists should identify and explore with clients the particular form or forms of clients' disrespect for animals and the underlying dynamics. Some clients give absolute priority to human needs and fail to acknowledge the needs and interests of animals. Supported by most laws, they treat animals as property whose value is limited to their market value. Others see animals as beings to be controlled and relationships with them are limited to training and discipline. Still others treat animals as an extension of the self, rather than distinct entities with their own interests and life. A common example of this is found in dog-fighting subcultures where the esteem of the individual is invested in the prowess and courage of his or her dog. Aside from this narcissistic relationship, animal abuse may become a prescription for higher self-esteem. Through intimidating, humiliating, and abusive behavior toward animals, clients establish themselves as "top dog."

Here is the first of two exercises involving respect.

Exercise: Teaching Respect

For most clients, this exercise should begin with focusing on a relationship with another human. The therapist asks clients to identify a person who has shown genuine respect for them, if possible someone in their family of origin. Since many clients confuse respect with power or prestige, it is essential that the therapist clarify that respect is the acknowledgement of another individual's worth. By asking clients to recall a situation in which they were shown respect, the therapist hopes to establish a model of a respectful relationship which can then be applied to human-animal relationships.

Some clients become defensive and respond to discussions about respect with a boastful review of their accomplishments and conquests. Others can recall few, if any, occasions when they felt acknowledged or valued by others. Therapists can circumvent these evasions by asking who cared for the client when they were sick or "down and out."

Therapists can begin this exercise by saying:

> Respect is a basic ingredient in any relationship with another living being — human and animal. We all deserve respect. And we all feel good when we receive respect. Think back to a time when you felt you received respect from another person. Tell me about it. What did that person do? How did you feel about it?

The goal is for the therapist to assist clients in recalling an occasion when they were respected and then in amplifying the feelings surrounding that event: How was the respect shown? How do they think the person felt when showing respect? How did it feel to be respected? How did it affect their sense of self-worth?

Using this as a model, the therapist then asks the client to imagine what it would feel like to show respect for an animal and then to imagine how the animal would feel when he or she was shown respect. This can be done virtually or in the presence of an animal in the session. In any case, the therapist asks clients to describe in detail an interaction in which they felt respect for an animal, again, both the feelings of respecting and of being respected. Once this has been explored, clients can be asked to compare this kind of interaction to their own treatment of animals, both nonabusive and abusive.

Homework Assignment

If direct interaction with an animal in the session is not possible, choose a setting in which clients can observe the interactions of people and animals under proper supervision—a humane society, a dog obedience class, or the office of a veterinarian. Ask clients to choose an interaction in which the person respected the animal. Describe the interaction in detail, including the effect it had on the animal and how it exemplified a respectful stance toward the animal. Again, the therapist can ask clients to compare this respectful interaction with their own treatment of animals: How are they alike? How are they different?

Exercise: Respecting Differences

Although always colored by our own experience, through empathy we have access to the experience of other individuals, including animals. The *Teaching Respect* exercise builds on the similarities between humans and other animals—like us they have interests, they can feel, and they can act autonomously. The present exercise, "respecting differences," features the recognition of the differences between humans and animals and, generally, between different species of animals. It can be a complementary or an alternative way to help clients establish respect for others.

This exercise also provides another context in which the therapist can explore with clients the issue of their views of nonhuman animals. As is the case with domestic violence conflict, male perpetrators, may perceive their partners as inferior beings with the limited role of servant or sex object. This is even more often the case in animal abuse. In the literature on the ethics of our treatment of animals, this belief is referred to as "speciesism" (Ryder 1975).

The exercise challenges clients' beliefs that humans are the center of the universe and that other animals have value only to the degree that they serve human interests. The "respecting difference" exercise extends the commonly recognized value of diversity within human cultures to the diversity across species. Although humans and animals both feel pain and pleasure, they also have very different needs and interests, and they can be respected and appreciated for who they are.

In the initial use of this exercise, therapists could ask clients to select a species other than the one or ones that they abused. Clients are presented with the following scenario:

> Imagine what it would be like if you and a cat were treated exactly alike: You lived in a similar space, were provided with the same food and the same limited comforts, and had the same limited access to the outdoors. How would you feel about this?

If clients object to the idea of being treated like an animal, the therapist might ask: "Why does this situation seem ridiculous to you? Now, take this situation from the animal's point of view. How would it be for him or her?" As the client responds, the therapist should coach the client to think about the particular needs and interests of this animal and animals of other species. For example, cats need to scratch, dogs sleep more than humans, and horses need to exercise. The point is to stimulate a discussion about the differences among animals including humans that emphasizes the value of diversity and of tolerance of that diversity. What does the client think of the fact that there are millions of different species? Does the client believe that some animals are more important than others? Explore the possibility that clients might have harmed an animal based on a misconception that the animal's needs, interests, and capabilities were the same as theirs.

Homework Assignment
Ask the client to select an animal and learn about that animal's habits, requirements, interests, and capabilities. The therapist can offer the client direction on where to find the necessary reference materials. It is up to the therapist whether to begin with an animal of the species that clients abused or start with another species and move to that one later.

3.4.2 Nurturance

Like accommodation, discussed earlier in the section on compassion, nurturing is an interpersonal skill through which clients recognize and meet the needs of others, including animals. Clients who have abused animals may not realize that other animals need nurturance and, in fact, can and do reciprocate by providing nurturance to people. The purpose of this exercise is to introduce clients to the rewards inherent in caring for another being, including animals, and to the possibility of having some of their own needs for nurturance or support be met by animals.

With primary interests in controlling animals' behavior to reinforce their own dominance and power or to control the behavior of other people, animal abusers often find it difficult to nurture. Although abusers may receive some gratification from exerting control over animals, they fail to realize the benefits derived from nurturing and, in turn, being nurtured by animals and often, as well, other people.

The therapist should educate clients about the demonstrated benefits of companion animal relationships which include advantages in physical health (lower blood pressure, faster recovery from illnesses) and mental health (less stress, more social engagement). For a review and critique of this literature, see Herzog (1991, 2011).

In the other direction, the therapist should point out various ways in which people can receive emotional gratification through nurturing and caring for animals. Ask clients to recall an individual who nurtured them and/or to create an image of a kindly, capable caretaker. What attitudes does this nurturing caretaker possess? How does he or she treat animals? Next, instruct clients to imagine that they are that caretaker. How would they treat animals? What would be different about their relationship? Ask the client to identify or imagine a specific situation in which he or she nurtures an animal and to explore how the animal responds to this caretaking. How would the client feel in the role of caretaker? If the therapist feels clients are ready to do so, ask them to compare that relationship to the relationship they had and could have had with the animal they abused.

Homework Assignment

As in the previous exercise on flexibility, if providing an animal in the therapy is not feasible, therapists can help clients arrange for direct experiences with animals (in a shelter, sanctuary, or dog training class where adequate supervision is available) to practice nurturing. Ask the client to reflect on this experience of nurturance and to describe it briefly, paying attention to what the client and the animal were each feeling during the nurturing activity.

3.5 Complementary Approaches

The approaches and types of interventions that we have adapted and included earlier in this section on intervention are cognitive behaviorism, attachment theory, psychodynamic therapy, and motivational interviewing. Here we provide a brief survey of other approaches which therapists can adapt for the treatment of this varied population. Therapists can adapt and emphasize their own favored approach to AniCare; alternatively, therapists can adapt or use the AniCare Approach adjunctively in their preferred approach.

As with many psychological problems (depression, anxiety disorders, and interpersonal violence), there are many pathways to or risk factors associated with animal abuse. We have discussed faulty attachment as one risk factor. Although developed to deal with other behavioral problems, some of the approaches described here are useful for their possible insights into other pathways to and/or conditions that can predispose an individual to or sustain the behavior of animal abuse.

3.5.1 Problem-Solving Therapy

Arguably, one predisposing and sustaining condition is poor problem-solving ability and the negative views of self that often accompany it. Although this intervention strategy and the one we have presented under the heading "interpersonal skills" have much in common and both are offshoots of cognitive behavioral therapy, problem-solving therapy is distinctive enough to be considered as a complementary approach to AniCare.

The skill component of problem-solving therapy is generally presented to clients in the form of several steps: (1) problem definition and selection, (2) generation of alternative solutions, (3) assessment and selection of solution, and (4) implementation and verification of solution. See the AniCare Child Handbook for a version of these steps in the context of the treatment of juveniles who abuse animals (Shapiro et al. 2014, pp. 55–58).

However, beyond the occasional use of this skill, proponents of problem-solving therapy maintain that problem-solving can be an effective way of living in the world more generally (Nezu et al. 2013). According to these investigators, adopting a "positive problem orientation" (p. 284) involves a general attitude or worldview, as well as a particular set of skills. Therapists can help their clients learn to approach situations in everyday life as possible problems and, as importantly, to develop confidence that they can solve them. Clients learn to define and identify problems in their daily dealings with others and the world. A problem is defined broadly to refer to any situation where there is a real or perceived discrepancy between the situational demands and the individual's ability to cope with it, both practically and emotionally. Clients gain confidence through the exploration of any feelings of inadequate self-efficacy and through learning and effectively implementing the skill.

Therapists can readily apply this intervention strategy, both the skill and the general orientation, to situations that have given rise to animal abuse. Particularly in regard to the former, therapists should consider the most effective presentation sequence of the three variables discussed earlier: subjects of the relationship, valence of the content, and directness of the presence of animals.

As exercises supplementing the learning of the steps in the skill, therapists can ask clients to identify examples of interactions in which a person (1) failed to recognize or identify a problem, (2) was faced with a problem and showed poor use of problem-solving skills, and (3) demonstrated good use of problem-solving skills. Eventually, therapists can help clients understand the role that the absence of a positive problem orientation played in the onset of their abusive behavior toward animals.

3.5.2   Trauma-Focused Therapy

Traumatic experiences have been identified as a risk factor for later psychological disorders, notably posttraumatic stress disorder. Accordingly, therapies have developed that focus on the treatment of trauma-based conditions (Courtois and Ford 2009). Traumatic events include being the victim of or witnessing interpersonal violence or sexual abuse, as well as natural or man-made disasters. Traumatic conditions can be caused by single or multiple events or prolonged exposure to insidious threats.

People suffer anxiety, depression, and intrusive memories in the aftermath of traumatic experiences and often constrict their lives to avoid any situations that might evoke memories of their trauma or become emotionally numbed. Among the behavioral manifestations of traumatized individuals are aggression, excessive temper, and acting-out behaviors.

In the present context of working with adults who abuse animals, it is notable that one of the acting-out behaviors is imitation of the traumatic event (National Child Traumatic Stress 2015). This suggests that a subpopulation of adults who abuse animals may have been traumatized by witnessing animal abuse. Studies show that witnessing animal abuse is a risk factor for later psychological problems (Gullone and Robertson 2008; Thompson and Gallone 2006). Boat (2014) has argued that acts of cruelty to animals perpetrated or witnessed in childhood should be considered a trauma to be included in the constellation of more widely accepted

Adverse Childhood Experiences (ACES). For some children, perpetration of animal abuse is a way to reduce the distress of traumatic memories. It is likely that the experience of such events is also a risk factor for animal abuse in adulthood. In addition, given the correlation between violence toward humans and animal abuse, pathways and risk factors leading to one may very well lead to the other.

For these reasons, assessment of clients should include taking a history of direct exposure to traumatic events, as well as the witnessing of events that might have been traumatic ("vicarious traumatization").

Therapists using a trauma-based approach expose clients to the originating traumatic object or situation through imagined scenarios or through actual direct exposure ("in vivo") to the originating trauma. This intervention might be an effective complement to AniCare interventions in clients with a history of exposure to traumatic events.

In addition, the direct or indirect presence of animals may be therapeutic for such clients. A number of preliminary studies show that animal-assisted interventions can be beneficial in the treatment of clients suffering from traumatic events (Yorke et al. 2008; Lefkowitz et al. 2005).

3.5.3 Narrative Therapy

Social scientists have demonstrated that a key component of personal identity is how people describe themselves (Gergen and Gergen 1984). Identities are not somehow direct representations of the events in people's lives; rather, they are shaped by the narrative or story that people tell others. How people present themselves to other people, their "social construction," is a primary way they maintain and develop their identity or self-concept.

Narrative psychotherapy takes advantage of the formative role of these self-accounts by working with clients to reconstruct their story (White 2007). White and Epston (1990) argue that putting clients' problems in the context of a self-narrative allows clients to "externalize" or get some distance from them. Therapists, then, serve as collaborators or coauthors and can suggest alternative viewpoints in the construction of the story. In this way, a self-defining story is developed that integrates the client's presenting problems into a coherent story that is socially acceptable and promotes positive self-esteem.

As we have described, adults who abuse animals often present with a justificatory story which denies any wrongdoing and/or any responsibility or accountability for the abusive behavior. This is an opening for the use of narrative therapy. However, it is not clear whether the collaborative role between therapist and client requisite to this work assumes a good working relationship or is a way to achieve such. It may be that the externalization of the presenting problem itself reduces anxiety and defensiveness and allows collaborative work on exploring alternative perspectives. On the other hand, it may be that the framing of the story as an externalization reinforces the position of refusing responsibility and self-blame. Again here, narrative-based therapists would suggest that the initial separation of the problem from clients by locating it in their story provides an opening for an alternative story in which assuming responsibility is an acceptable component.

More generally, through the narrative approach and their collaboration in its construction, therapists can reframe the story from a focus on the problem and its denial to a focus on solutions. *What could the character in this story have done differently?*

Conclusion

In the intervention section of this handbook, we have addressed the complex and varied presentations that involve the behavior of animal abuse. While theoretically eclectic, we have mostly stayed on the ground, providing a set of practical, nuts-and-bolts interventions. They are meant to be tools applicable in cases where the behavior of animal abuse is one of the several presenting problems as well as where it is the primary problem. Finally, we have indicated how therapists may adopt the AniCare Approach *in toto* or adapt it piecemeal to complement other approaches.

Appendices

4

4.1 Appendix A: Supplementary Cases

The following case thumbnails are based on actual scenarios but have been modified to assure anonymity and for pedagogical purposes. The set has been compiled to illustrate the broad range of presentations of adults who have abused animals. We have tried to incorporate some of the variables discussed in the text, organized here by relevant categories:

- Demographics—age, gender, ethnicity
- Form of abuse—egregious harm, killing, neglect, hoarding (two types), dog fighting, sexual abuse, subcultural based
- Perpetrator dynamics or personality variables—instrumental or expressive, animal punishment or partner retaliatory, callous or sensitive, externalized or internalized
- Comorbidity—psychopathy, addiction, psychosis, post-traumatic stress disorder, depression
- Individual or group perpetration
- Association with violence to humans—domestic violence or elder abuse link
- Attachment history—negative or positive
- Family history—negative or positive
- Attitude to counseling—compliant/resistant/defensive

Name: Roy
Age: 45
Gender: Male
Ethnicity: Caucasian

Referral With two other men, Roy shot and killed five cows and seriously injured two others, following an unsuccessful attempt to "get their deer." They killed the cows over a period of 3 weeks before they were apprehended. In addition to being

© Springer International Publishing Switzerland 2016
K. Shapiro, A.J.Z. Henderson, *The Identification, Assessment, and Treatment of Adults Who Abuse Animals: The AniCare Approach*,
DOI 10.1007/978-3-319-27362-4_4

required to compensate the farmers for their cattle, Roy was sentenced to a fine of $1000, 9 months in jail, and required to complete a 20-week counseling program as a condition of his probation.

Social and Educational Background Roy has been married and divorced twice. He lives with his sister, her husband, and children. In addition to his sister, Roy has an older brother who is divorced and has two DUI arrests.

Roy's parents are deceased. His father did not abuse his children; however, he was a harsh disciplinarian, often using corporal punishment as a means to control or change his children's behavior. The mother did not discipline the children, but would defer to the father. Although the father did not strike the mother, he dominated her and the children. Roy's family occasionally attended the local Baptist church. Other than that, the family did not participate in any community activities.

Roy has a high school education, plus 6 weeks of trade school. He belongs to a social group of men who play pool and hunt together. When a juvenile, Roy was apprehended for shoplifting once and for disorderly conduct another time. In both cases, he was with two of his friends when he committed these offenses.

History of Companion Animals Roy's family had a number of dogs, all used for hunting. The dogs were kept outside of the house in runs or tethered and did not enter the family's home.

Self-Presentation Roy and his sister's family were bewildered and angry by his conviction. While they acknowledge the fairness in being required to compensate the farmers for their economic losses, they "didn't see what the big fuss was about animals that were going to be killed anyway." Roy stated that "this is just another case of the government sticking their noses in where it doesn't belong."

Name: Harry
Age: 59
Gender: Male
Ethnicity: Caucasian

Referral Harry was charged with cruelty to animals resulting in death. Harry lives on his five-acre ranch and became annoyed when his neighbor's small dog continually yelped at him as he was mowing his lawn. He shot the dog two times with his pellet gun. He stated that this dog had been digging in his yard for the past 5 years and that he had had enough. He did not know that the dog had died until 2 days later.

Social and Educational Background Harry's mother was schizophrenic and hospitalized when he was approximately 3 years old. He lived with his aunt and uncle, and his sister lived with another aunt. He did not know why his father was unable to care for them and they were sent to live with relatives. His father remarried and his stepmother had four additional children. His stepmother and biological father did their "fair share of drinking." His biological sister committed suicide by "torching" herself. When disciplined, which was seldom, it was with a belt. He has been married for 29 years and 7 months. He has two children, a boy and girl, and they will shortly be moving closer to him. His wife died in 2002 from leukemia.

Harry graduated from high school with average grades and joined the National Guard where he served for 6 years and 6 months. He completed carpenter training and worked for 30 years with one company before retiring.

History of Companion Animals   Harry had no pets growing up. He has a dog now and does not believe in being cruel. He denied doing anything wrong because he had repeatedly alerted his neighbor to the dog's problematic behavior, and was unaware until recently that the dog had in fact died.

Self-Presentation   Harry presented as cooperative and reflected a desire to appear in a favorable light. His affect and speech were flat, and his mood apathetic. When talking about his own dog, he seemed to lack any expression of affection and/or sincere warmth. He stated that "he had had enough of this yelping dog." He said that he was sorry but his affect lacked empathy or authenticity.

Name: Polly
Age: 52
Gender: Female
Ethnicity: Caucasian

Referral   Neighbors complained to the authorities of a terrible stench coming from Polly's home. When the authorities opened the garage door, they found over 25 dogs and cats. Most of the animals were dead or beyond help, feces were everywhere, and the animals looked dazed. The animals made no responses when the authorities placed them in their truck. Polly was charged with animal cruelty for failing to provide food, housing, and veterinary care.

Social and Educational Background   Polly is a divorced woman who lives alone. Her two adult children live in another state. She reports a positive childhood experience with her parents who cared for her and her two sisters. Poly is the oldest sibling. Both parents are now deceased. She was divorced when her two daughters were 6 and 7 years of age. She had good grades in high school and completed 3 years of college in a program for medical librarians. She works full time in the local library. She has a very limited social life.

History of Companion Animals   Polly and her sisters had cats whom they dearly loved and cared for. There is no history of neglect or of legal difficulties.

Self-Presentation   Polly reported that she was struggling to care for so many animals but felt compelled to do so when the animal shelter asked her to foster parent. She could not deny these helpless unwanted animals, and did not want to see them euthanized. She felt she had few alternatives. She had no money for dog or cat food, her house was not selling, and she wanted to be closer to her daughters. She could not understand what harm she had done. She left what food and water she could and provided numerous litter boxes. Polly stated, "I did what I could to save these animals and I should not be charged with such a terrible crime."

Name: Sally
Age: 62
Gender: Female
Ethnicity: Hispanic

Referral An emaciated cat was found outside of Sally's apartment, leading to an investigation by the local animal control officer. Sally had been out of town for a couple of days and had been unable to retrieve the cat before leaving. She has received an eviction notice for failure to maintain the apartment, which is covered with animal excrement. Sally was charged with neglect of ten cats, three dogs, and one bird. Complaints of animal noises and odor had been received from neighbors of Sally's two previous residences in the same town.

Social and Educational Background Sally is a single woman living alone. She has been unemployed for 10 years and receives Medicare support. Her father and mother divorced when she was a teenager. She has one older sister who is unmarried, works full-time for an ad agency, and with whom Sally occasionally gets together on holidays. She graduated from nursing school and worked in a suburban hospital.

History of Companion Animals Her mother had a number of animals and, following her death, Sally, at that time in her 20s, continued living in her family home. It is likely that she has lived with a large collection of animals since her 40s.

Self-Presentation Sally appears to be in good health but has rotting teeth. She denies there is a problem and feels that city officials just want to control her valuable animals. She believes that people may be trying to poison her animals. She avoids veterinary care for her animals as she does not trust the competency of treatment provided.

Name: John
Age: 34
Gender: Male
Ethnicity: Caucasian

Referral John "exercised" his dog by chaining him to the back of his car while he drove it. The dog died in the incident. John was found guilty of cruelty to animals and served time in prison.

Social and Educational Background John lives with his wife, Mary, their three children, John, Jr., Steven, and Theresa. John works as a loan officer in a bank and Mary is a homemaker. Their 6-year-old son is repeating kindergarten. His teacher reports that he has difficulty concentrating and is not ready for first grade.

John's family of origin consisted of his parents and two younger brothers. His father was an insurance agent and his mother worked in the home. John's father had been arrested on two occasions for assaulting his wife, who later withdrew the charges. One of John's younger brothers joined the military and the other, who is estranged from the family, became an environmental activist.

John earned a bachelor's degree from a local college. He is a reliable employee at the bank, and he and his family attend a church in the community. John and his family attend some of the church social events. John also belongs to a men's bowling league.

History of Companion Animals   John's family of origin kept a number of dogs, but no dog remained in the family for more than a year.

Self-Presentation   John clearly resented his conviction and having to attend counseling. He strongly denied responsibility for wrongdoing. In presenting an account of the incident with his dog, he was withholding and minimizing. His cognitive style is literal and rigid.

Name: Jerry
Age: 19
Gender: Male
Ethnicity: African-American

Referral   Jerry killed his girlfriend's pet rabbit with a baseball bat. Jerry was sentenced to 2 years probation, 1 year suspended jail sentence, prohibitions against having animals during the 2 years, and contact with the girlfriend. He was required to attend and complete AniCare treatment.

Social and Educational Background   Jerry lives with his parents and works at a sporting goods store. He has an older brother who is in the armed forces and is stationed abroad. His parents both work full-time, father in a factory and mother as a housekeeper in a hotel. Jerry has been seeing his current girlfriend for 2 years. They have broken up and reconciled several times. This is Jerry's first serious relationship.

Jerry is a high school graduate. He was on the baseball team and played first string his junior and senior years. He was charged with DUI when he was 16 and required to complete a diversion program for substance abusers.

History of Companion Animals   Jerry's family always had pets during his childhood, both cats and dogs. Jerry had responsibilities for these animals—feeding and walking in the case of the dogs. Currently, the family has one dog and one cat.

Self-Presentation   Jerry resents having to undergo psychological treatment. He is of average intelligence but not psychologically minded. When asked about his feelings about killing the rabbit, he states that he misses seeing his girlfriend.

Name: Ted
Age: 38
Gender: Male
Ethnicity: Caucasian

Referral Ted was convicted of animal cruelty for poisoning four feral cats. He claims that the cats were keeping him up at night and he couldn't sleep. He has a chronic problem with insomnia.

Social and Educational Background Ted completed an associates' degree in computing at the local community college. He works as a computer programmer and is competent at his work. He had a girlfriend when he was in his mid-20s. They lived together for 1 year and then she moved out of state. He was very disappointed when the relationship broke up. He has lived alone since then and indicates that he does not go out much and does not have much confidence in forming relationships with women or men.

History of Companion Animals When he was growing up, Ted had a dog that he spent a lot of time with and cared for a great deal.

Self-Presentation "I guess I was feeling at rock bottom. It was 3 o'clock in the morning and I hadn't slept well for days. And those cats were making that hollering noise—it is spooky. After I decided to poison them I guess I felt a kind of "rush"… At least I was doing something about a problem. It's weird, but I felt energized in a way."

Name: Aaron
Age: 22
Gender: Male
Ethnicity: African-American

Referral Aaron was ordered by the courts to undergo counseling when he was convicted of animal cruelty. He beat his own dog, Lady, with a hammer, nearly killing her, when she ran after a squirrel in the park instead of coming to him when he called her.

Social and Educational Background Aaron lives with his parents and three siblings in an urban housing project. He gets along with his family and with other members of the extended family that live nearby. He has a girlfriend. After completing high school, he got a job at a car-rental agency where he has worked for 3 years.

History of Companion Animals When Aaron was in high school, he convinced his parents for the first time to get a companion animal. They adopted a dog from the local shelter and Aaron trained her and spent a great deal of time with her.

Self-Presentation Aaron described how he hung around with other kids who had dogs and trained them. He was known as a good dog trainer and Lady had let him down in front of his friends by disobeying him. "I get mad when I think of her 'dissing' me that way, but I guess she probably didn't mean to do it."

Name: Abby
Age: 20
Gender: Female
Ethnicity: Caucasian

Referral Abby was charged with animal abuse for allegedly encasing her boyfriend's dog in tape and attaching him upside down to the refrigerator.

Social and Educational Background Abby spent the first year of her life with her single mother. When her mother entered treatment for drug abuse, she was moved into foster care. She had three sets of foster parents until she left home at 16. She completed one semester at a community college and then took a job as a waitress.

History of Companion Animals The second set of foster parents where Abby lived during her early teens had a cat. Abby tolerated the cat but had no relationship with him.

Self-Presentation She claims that the dog bit her and that her boyfriend promised to get rid of him but did not. She described how she planned the taping by acquiring tape and scissors. She does not seem contrite about the treatment of the dog.

Name: Doug
Age: 30
Gender: Male
Ethnicity: Caucasian

Referral Investigating neighbors' complaints of a dog howling through the night, police found an emaciated black lab chained in the backyard. Doug was charged with gross neglect under an anti-cruelty statute.

Social and Educational Background Doug's father died when Doug was 14 years old. He has one older sister who has serious health problems. Recently, when his mother broke her hip and became non-ambulatory, Doug returned to the family home to care for her. According to his mother, he asked her to sign over the house to him and she refused because of his poor work and money management history.

Until her accident, the dog was well cared for and provided major companionship for his mother. However, Doug has consigned the dog to the backyard where he howls and cries to be let in.

Doug has had various unskilled and semi-skilled jobs, usually being fired for poor performance—arguing with staff or customers. He was arrested twice for getting into fights, but the charges were dropped.

History of Companion Animals Doug reports no history of companion animals as a child or adult.

Self-Presentation Doug brusquely denied any wrong doing, claiming that the dog was well cared for and couldn't come in the house as he was underfoot. He vowed he would seek legal counsel and fight against the charges.

Name: Alan
Age: 28
Gender: Male
Ethnicity: Caucasian

Referral Alan was referred to an AniCare provider following lengthy participation and compliance with substance abuse treatment. The presenting problem was that Alan was neglecting his dog. He would regularly tie the dog outside of bars for long periods of time without shelter or water. On one occasion, the dog was attacked by a feral dog and badly injured.

Social and Educational Background Alan's father abandoned the family in response to his wife's excessive drinking. An only child, he was raised by his mother with occasional assistance from her sister and brother-in-law who lived nearby.

Once he reached his teen years, Alan spent very little time at home, preferring to socialize and party with his friends. He dropped out of high school in his junior year without completing his vocational training as an auto mechanic. He is currently employed as an assistant mechanic in a gas station.

History of Companion Animals Alan had a close attachment to a dog during his middle school years and was the primary caretaker. The dog was euthanized following a stroke.

Self-Presentation Alan presents that he is in the early stages of recovery from addiction to alcohol and that he is confident that he can stay sober. It is not clear that he understands the seriousness and recalcitrance of the addiction. He claims to be contrite about his irresponsible treatment and subsequent injury of his dog.

Name: Sheldon
Age: 27
Gender: Male
Ethnicity: Caucasian

Referral Sheldon was charged with animal abuse for stalking a number of dogs and having sex with them.

Social and Educational Background   Sheldon was raised on a farm with his parents and five siblings. They all joined in the work of the farm and seemed to get along. One of his female siblings claims that when he was 13 he tried to stab her with a knife. Two of the siblings joined the army; the others remained in the area working on farms and local businesses.

Sheldon never liked school but did complete high school. He has been in and out of mental institutions through his 20s.

History of Companion Animals   Sheldon and his male siblings would occasionally have sex with some of the farm animals. He also admits catching stray dogs and cats and sexually abusing them and sometimes killing them. He was caught putting the family cat into a microwave oven and sent for treatment.

Self-Presentation   Sheldon describes himself as antisocial and claims that he is an animal trapped in a human's body. He states, "when I am angry or upset, I feel better in the company of an animal."

Name: Sam
Age: 20
Gender: Male
Ethnicity: Caucasian

Referral   Following his conviction for animal abuse, Sam was referred by the court for psychological evaluation. He and a friend set fire to a kitten that then ran under a car causing the car to blow up.

Social and Educational Background   His mother describes Sam as difficult to manage as an infant. As a child he was easily bored and hot-tempered, often feeling like he was mistreated by his parents. His father was physically abusive to his mother— he once threatened her with a gun and, on another occasion, injured her seriously enough to require hospitalization. He is an alcoholic and also uses pot and cocaine.

Sam had to repeat the fifth grade and once was suspended for stealing from another student in middle school. He did graduate from high school.

History of Companion Animals   Sam had several animals in succession during his childhood, none of them lasting very long. Two dogs, in particular, were a source of comfort to him in times of stress. They did not have cats as his father did not like them.

Self-Presentation   Sam showed mild disorganization in interviews and reports that he gets upset when stressed. He showed little empathy for the kitten.

4.2   Appendix B: Screening Instrument

Animal-Related Experiences

Screening Questions for Adults*

1. **Do you have a pet or pets now?**   Y _____ N _____
   How many?

   a. Dog(s) _____   f. Turtles, snakes, lizards, insects, etc. _____

   b. Cat(s) _____   g. Rabbits, hamsters, mice, guinea pigs, gerbils _____

   c. Bird(s) _____   h. Wild animals (describe) _____

   d. Fish(es) _____   i. Other (describe)_____

   e. Horse(s) _____

2. **Did you ever have any pets?**   Y _____ N _____
   How many?

   a. Dog(s) _____   f. Turtles, snakes, lizards, insects, etc. _____

   b. Cat(s) _____   g. Rabbits, hamsters, mice, guinea pigs, gerbils _____

   c. Bird(s) _____   h. Wild animals (describe) _____

   d. Fish(es) _____

   e. Horse(s) _____

3. **Has your pet ever been hurt?**   Y _____ N _____

   What happened? (describe) _____
   _____

   ___ a. Accidental? (hit by car, attacked by another animal, fell, ate something, etc.)

   ___ b. Deliberate? (kicked, punched, thrown, not fed, etc.)

4. **Have you ever felt afraid for your pet or worried about bad things happening to your pet?**   Y___N _____

   (describe) _____
   _____

   Are you worried now?   Y _____ N _____

5. **Have you ever lost a pet you really cared about? (e.g. Was given away, ran away, died or was some how**
   killed?)   Y _____ N _____

   What kind of pet? _____   If your pet died, was the death:

   ___ a. Natural (old age, illness, euthanized)   _____b. Accidental (hit by car)

   ___c. Deliberate (strangled, drowned)   ____d. Cruel or violent (e.g. pet was tortured)

   What happened? _____ __
   _____
   _____

   Was the death or loss used to punish you or make you do something?   Y _____ N _____

   How difficult was the loss for you?

   ___ a. Not difficult   _____b. Somewhat difficult   _____c. Very difficult

   How much does it bother you now?

   ___ a. Not at all   _____b. Somewhat   _____c. A lot

   How did people react/what did they tell you after you lost your pet?

   ___ a. Supportive   _____b. Said it was your fault   _____c. Punished you   _____d. Other _____

   How old were you?

   ___ a. Under age 6   _____b. 6-12 years   _____c. Teenager   _____d. Adult

6. Have you ever <u>seen</u> some one hurt an animal or pet?   Y_____N_____

How many?

a. Dog(s) _____   f. Turtles, snakes, lizards, insects, etc. _____

b. Cat(s) _____   g. Rabbits, hamsters, mice, guinea pigs, gerbils _____

c. Bird(s) _____   h. Wild animals (describe) _____

d. Fish(es) _____   i. Other (describe) _____

e. Horse(s) _____

What did they do?

___ a. Drowned   ___ g. Burned

___ b. Hit, beat, kicked   _____h. Starved or neglected

___ c. Stoned   ___ i. Trapped

___ d. Shot (BB gun, bow & arrow) _____ j. Had sex with the animal

___ e. Strangled   ___ k. Other (describe) _____

___ f. Stabbed

Was it _____a. Accidental?   _____b. Deliberate?   ____c. Coerced?

How old were you? (mark all that apply)

___ a. Under age 6   ____b. 6-12 years   _____c. Teenager   _____d. Adult

Were they hunting the animal for food or sport?   Y_____N_____

Did anyone know they did this?   Y_____N_____

What happened afterwards?_____

7. Have <u>you</u> ever hurt an animal or pet?   Y_____N_____

How many?

a. Dog(s) _____   f. Turtles, snakes, lizards, insects, etc. _____

b. Cat(s) _____   g. Rabbits, hamsters, mice, guinea pigs, gerbils _____

c. Bird(s) _____   h. Wild animals (describe) _____

d. Fish(es) _____   i. Other (describe) _____

e. Horse(s) _____

What did you do?

___ a. Drowned   ___ g. Burned

___ b. Hit, beat, kicked   _____h. Starved or neglected

___ c. Stoned   ___ i. Trapped

___ d. Shot (BB gun, bow & arrow) _____ j. Had sex with the animal

___ e. Strangled   ___ k. Other (describe) _____

___ f. Stabbed

Was it _____a. Accidental?   _____b. Deliberate?   _____c. Coercive?

How old were you? (mark all that apply)

___ a. Under age 6   ____b. 6-12 years   _____c. Teenager   _____d. Adult

Were they hunting the animal for food or sport?   Y_____N_____

Did anyone know they did this?   Y_____N_____

What happened afterwards?_____

*Adapted from Boat (1999) Abuse of children and abuse of animals: using the links to inform child assessment and protection. In: Ascione and Arkow (eds) Child abuse, domestic violence, and animal abuse: Linking the circles of compassion for prevention and intervention. Purdue University Press, West Lafayette, pp 83–100.

4.3   Appendix C: History

Psychological and Social History*

Name: _____   Today's Date: _____

Family of Origin History

How many brothers and sisters do you have and where are you in the birth order?   _____

To whom in your family do you feel closest?   _____

Were your parents separated or divorced? _____How old were you? _____

With whom did you live with when you were growing up?   _____

How did your parents get along with each other?   _____

Did you have a relationship with both parents?   _____

Describe your family and childhood.   _____

Has anyone physically or emotionally abused you?   _____Who? _____

Did anyone in your family have a problem with drugs?   _____   Alcohol? _____

Circle which person(s):   Dad   Mom   brothers/sisters   aunts/uncles   grandparents

Do your parents or grandparents have mental health problems?   _____

If so, what kind? _____

As a child, did you have companion animals?   _____

If so, what happened to them? _____

How often did you move? _____Have you been neglected or abandoned by your parents? _____

Has anyone close to you died?   _____Yes   _____No

Relationship of that person to you: _____Cause of death:_____

Were either of your parents in the military?   _____

Relationship History

Are you currently involved in a relationship?   _____Yes   _____No

If yes, how long? _____

Describe your partner _____

Describe your partner's attitude toward you   _____

How do you feel about your partner?   _____

Have you ever thought your partner was cheating? _____

Have you ever followed your partner or "checked up on the partner" to see what he/she was doing?   _____

Do you think that you are jealous or possessive?_____

How many serious relationships have you had? _____

Have you had an affair or cheated on someone?_____

How long was the longest relationship that you have had? _____

Have you ever been divorced or separated?_____How many times? _____

Do you prefer sexual relationships with _____women?_____men?_____both?

List your children and step children. Put a check mark next to those not currently living with you. Name

Age   Name   Age

_____   _____

_____   _____

_____   _____

_____   _____

Education and Employment History

What was the highest grade you completed in school?   _____

Did you graduate from high school? _____What year? _____

If no, do you have a GED? _____Did you have learning difficulties in school?   ____

If yes, briefly explain? _____

Did you ever get into trouble in school?   _____

If yes, what happened? _____

Were you ever expelled or suspended from school? _____   If yes, for what? _____

Did you ever have problems with teachers or neighbors? _____

If yes, what happened? _____

What is your current employment? _____

How many jobs have you had in the past 5 years?   Have you ever had a problem with a boss? _____

Have you ever been fired? _____If yes, why? _____

How long have you been with your current job? _____

Legal History

How many times have you been arrested?_____Were you arrested as a juvenile?_____

Have you ever been arrested for domestic violence? _____How many times? _____

Have you ever been stopped for DWI or DUI? _____How many times? _____

Have you ever been arrested for a felony? _____

Please list the dates and reason for each arrest (regardless of conviction):

_____   _____
_____   _____
_____   _____

Do you currently have any outstanding warrants for your arrest? _____

Where? _____

Psychological History

Have you ever been in counseling or had to take classes?_____

Where? _____

For what? _____

Have you ever thought of suicide? _____   If yes, why? _____

When was the last time you thought about suicide? _____

Are you still thinking about it? _____What was your plan? _____

What is going on in your life when these thoughts occur? _____
_____

Have you ever had any of the following?

_____ Phobias (intense fear)   _____Delusions   _____Fear of going crazy

_____Panic attacks   _____ Hallucinations   _____Thoughts of killing someone

Violence Behavior Checklist and Assessment

Have you EVER done any of the following?

_____ Slapped, kicked, or shoved your partner   _____Blocked partner's path

_____ Slapped, kicked, or shoved children   _____ Indulged in mocking or name calling

_____ Hit your partner or children   _____ With held affection/sex

_____ Punched walls or broken personal property   _____Restrained partner/person

_____ Threatened to leave or divorce partner   _____Drunk or done drugs to relieve anger

_____ Become more angry as are sult of drinking or drugs

_____ Threatened someone with a weapon   _____ Threatened family, children, or pets

_____ Hurt an animal   _____ Except for hunting, killed an anim

_____ Had sex with your partner when he/she didn't want to

_____ Have you ever disciplined your children more than you meant to?

_____ What type of discipline do you use with your children?   _____

_____ Have you ever disciplined pets more than you meant to?

_____ Have you ever been abused _____ physically? _____ sexually? _____emotionally?

By whom? _____

Please check the experiences that you have witnessed:

_____ Parents hitting/hurting each other   _____ Parents hitting/hurting you

_____ Street crime   _____ War

Have you ever been in any fights (with friends, in bars, at school, etc.)?   _____

Drugs and Alcohol Use History

What drugs have you tried? Please check:

_____ (Pot) Marijuana   _____ Cocaine or crack   Downers

_____ Meth or Crystal Meth (Speed)   _____ LSD or PCP _____   Other _____   Inhalants

How old were you when you first drank alcohol? _____ Did drugs?

How often do you drink? _____   How often do you get high? _____

Have you ever gotten high on prescription drugs? _____ What drug(s)? _____

Have you ever gotten high on over the counter drugs? _____

When was the last time you drank or gothigh? _____

If we do a urine test today, will it be hot (positive)? _____

Have you ever felt you needed to cut down on your drinking or drug use? _____

If yes, briefly explain: _____

What was the longest period you have been able to remain drug/alcohol free? _____

How many times have you been to any of the following?

_____ Detox   _____ DUI classes

_____ Residential treatment   _____ Halfway House

List the programs or agencies in which you have been in treatment or classes for drug or alcohol: Program
                                                       Name   Year
_____
_____

Have you ever attended Alcoholics Anonymous or other 12 Step meetings? _____
Why? _____

How often have you had the following when you did drugs or drank?

_____ Memory loss or blackout   _____ Loss of control (drank or used more than you intended

_____ Personality changes   Please describe_____

_____ Stealing, sneaking or lying about, or hiding drugs or alcohol

Describe the consequences you have experienced from your drug or alcohol use

Legal consequences: _____

Personal consequences:_____

Medical Survey

How would you rate your health?   poor: _____   average: _____   excellent: _____

Are you currently under medical care? _____   For what reason? _____

Are you taking any medications or prescription drugs? _____   For what reason?

Name of your doctor: _____Last time you saw your doctor: _____

Have you ever had any of the following? Seizures _____   Heart problems _____

Learning disabilities _____   Head or brain injuries _____

FOR WOMEN: Are you pregnant? _____   If yes, are you receiving pre-natal care? _____

Military

Have you ever been in the military? _____   How long? _____

If yes, what kind of discharge do you have? _____

What is your veteran status? _____

Is there anything else we should know about you? _____

*Adapted from an intake protocol of the Aurora Center for Treatment, Aurora CO www.auroracentx.com\ (unpublished).

4.4   Appendix D: Animal Hoarding

4.4.1   What Is Animal Hoarding?

Animal hoarding poses a unique challenge to the treatment of animal abusers. Unlike other forms of deliberate animal cruelty where the perpetrator intends to harm animals, most animal hoarders firmly believe that they not only have the animals' best interests at heart but that they are the *only* ones who are capable of caring for them. With the notable exception of the "exploitative hoarder," discussed below, this belief persists in spite of palpable evidence to the contrary.

Animal hoarding has been defined as "…the accumulation of an unusually large number of animals, failure to provide adequate care and living environment for the animals, and impairment in health, safety, and social or occupational functioning" (Frost et al. 2011, p. 885). The possession of a large number of animals alone does not necessarily indicate the presence of a hoarding disorder, as breeders and trainers may have many animals but do so without the associated deteriorating care or any functioning impairments (Frost et al. 2011). The DSM-5 (American Psychiatric Association 2013) has given hoarding disorder (HD) its own unique classification, now distinct from obsessive-compulsive disorder, and includes animal hoarding as a condition associated with HD. However, the manual falls short of listing animal hoarding as a specific subtype. Since the DSM-5 criteria for HD do not specify what types of possessions are necessary for a diagnosis, and animals are legally considered possessions, the hoarding of animals, some argue, qualifies for a HD classification (Frost et al. 2015).

Although animal hoarders are typically found among the unemployed and socially isolated, animal hoarding does not appear to be bounded by social or economic class. Animal hoarding has been discovered among physicians, veterinarians, bankers, teachers, and college professors who often lead a double life (Arluke et al. 2002).

Because one animal hoarder may be responsible for the suffering of numerous, sometimes hundreds, of animals, animal hoarding is one of the most serious animal welfare issues faced by animal protection agencies. Recent epidemiological studies suggest that between 1 and 6 % of the US population meet the criteria for HD. making it one of the most frequent mental illnesses (Steketee and Frost 2014). The Hoarding of Animals Research Consortium (HARC, a group of researchers, collaborating to define and better understand animal hoarding) reports that there are approximately 3000–7000 new animal hoarding cases in the USA each year, with an estimated 250,000 animals being compromised (HARC 2015).

Almost any species of animal can be hoarded, and occasionally we see the hoarding of multiple species. Documented reports include companion animals such as dogs, cats, guinea pigs, rabbits, ferrets, and birds; farm animals such as horses, goats, sheep, chicken, and cattle; and even exotic and dangerous animals (HARC 2015). Hoarding cats fits the stereotype of the hoarder and cats are indeed the most commonly hoarded animal, undoubtedly because they are more easily obtained, cared for, and concealed and give rise to the stereotypical "crazy cat lady."

4.4.2   Characteristics of Animal Hoarding

In Patronek's (1999) groundbreaking study of 54 animal hoarding cases, the average number of hoarded animals was 39, though many cases had more than 100 animals living in deplorable conditions. The majority of situations were unsafe and unsanitary (77 %), had animal excrement in human living areas (69 %), and the presence of animal carcasses in the home (69 %). The majority of the cases (59.3 %) involved repeated visits to the same home, and the median number of visits per case was 7.5.

Subsequent research is consistent with Patronek's initial findings with animal hoarding cases typically involving older, socially isolated women, living with large numbers of sick, dying, and dead animals crammed into living spaces. Extreme squalor and highly unsanitary conditions appear in 70–90 % of hoarding cases, typified by homes contaminated with urine, feces, and dead and decomposing animals (Frost et al. 2015).

In a review of 71 animal hoarding cases from across the USA and Canada, HARC found that 83 % of the cases involved women. Most of these women (71 %) were widowed, divorced, or single. Fifty-three percent of the cases had other individuals living in the home, including children (5 %), elderly dependents (21 %), and disabled people (21 %). Nearly all of the homes (93 %) were extraordinarily unsanitary: most utilities and major appliances such as showers, heaters, stoves, toilets, and sinks were nonfunctional, most residences had several fire hazards, and 16 % had actually been condemned as unfit for habitation.

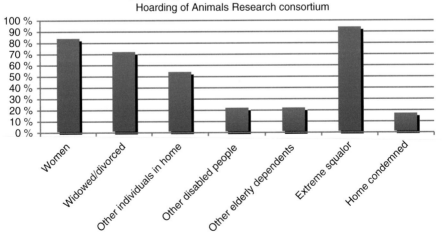

Characteristics of animal hoarders
Hoarding of Animals Research consortium

4.4.3 Characteristics Common to Object and Animal Hoarding

Maladaptive Beliefs As there are for people who collect or hoard inanimate objects, maladaptive beliefs about possessions seem to be common to animal hoarders, manifesting in a heightened sense of responsibility and exaggerated need for control (Tolin 2011). Perfectionist beliefs also make many hoarders reluctant to make decisions about bringing their chaos under control for fear that they will make the wrong decision (Tolin 2011). Poor executive function (attention difficulties, indecisiveness, difficulty with organization, and memory problems) typical of hoarders compounds the problem for effective intervention (Tolin 2011).

Excessive Acquisition Excessive acquisition can be conceived of as a behavioral disinhibition that may be impulsive in origin (positively reinforced behaviors because the acquisition makes the hoarder feel excited, clever, or good), or compulsive (acquisition operates as a negative reinforcer to reduce anxiety and discomfort from trying to refrain from acquiring) (Tolin 2011).

Clutter/Disorganization Living areas become so excessively cluttered as to become nonfunctional for their original intended use.

Difficulty Discarding Both object and animal hoarders experience distress or impaired functioning as a result of the hoarding and an extreme difficulty parting with possessions or animals. Object hoarders typically become distressed when anyone touches or displaces their objects. Similarly, many animal hoarders resist attempts of others to care for their animals, harboring a strong sense of distorted responsibility, an almost missionary zeal, that they alone have been called to save or rescue their animals.

Avoidance Tolin (2011) notes, that unlike obsessive-compulsive disorder (OCD), sufferers whose life is characterized by compulsive, time-consuming, rituals of repetitive behaviors, hoarders are characterized by what they do *not* do—they do not sort, nor organize, nor discard. Sorting and discarding is cognitively challenging as it runs counter to their deeply held beliefs about responsibility, control, and emotional attachment to their possessions.

Poor Insight Again, unlike OCD sufferers, both object and animal hoarders show surprising lack of awareness about the severity of their problem behaviors. Tolin (2011) reports that object hoarders typically did not recognize that they had a problem requiring treatment until 10 years after onset. He also reports that insight was negatively correlated with hoarders' self-reported level of distress (Tolin et al. 2010).

Limited Motivation Lack of insight may also be at the root of compromised motivation to change behavior. Hoarders are noted for poor homework adherence, inconsistent attendance in therapy, and high dropout rates (Tolin 2011). In a sample of hoarders who were reported to health departments because of excessive squalor, Frost et al. (2000) found that less than one-third were willing to cooperate with health officials to improve their unsanitary home environment.

4.4.4 Differences Between Object and Animal Hoarding

Who Hoards? Both object and animal hoarders are more likely to live alone and be socially isolated. However, animal hoarding is more common in women; object hoarding is more common in men (Frost et al. 2011).

Specificity of What Is Hoarded Object hoarders tend to hoard everything; it is rare for an object hoarder to limit collecting to a single category of objects (Frost et al. 2011). Research in the USA suggests that animal hoarders usually limit their collection to a single species, although this finding may not hold cross culturally. Multiple species-hoarding cases have been noted in Australia, for example, (Signal, personal communication).

Acquisition: Active vs. Passive Hoarding Object hoarders are more likely to be active acquirers of objects although some simply acquire objects through the normal accumulation of papers that are never sorted or discarded. Animal hoarders may be both active—purposefully and actively "rescuing" animals from shelters, online, or on the street, and even stealing animals, or passive—people bring animals to them, or animals accumulate due to failure to spay and neuter.

Squalor The inability to use living space because of disorganization and clutter is true of both object and animal hoarders. Both show extreme neglect of the home environment that results in an inability to manage the activities of daily living, including (in the case of animal hoarders) caring adequately for the animals. However, the unsanitary living conditions of animal hoarders, with feces, urine, and often dead animals present in their environment, is not typical of object hoarders. There is growing recognition of Diogenes syndrome (extreme squalor in some homes of the elderly—often as part of an overall dementia diagnoses). Some researchers are suggesting a sub-diagnosis particular to those hoarding animals—Noah syndrome—with psychosocial stress and extreme loneliness thought to be precipitating factors (Saldarriaga-Cantillo and Nieto 2015).

Difficulty Discarding Animal hoarders may experience an even greater distress about parting with their animals than object hoarders with their possessions. The parting may be more excruciating because of disturbed attachment relationships with the animals and hoarders' delusional beliefs about their sole responsibility toward their animals. This may account for the retention of deceased animals.

Poor Insight Lack of insight may be even more extreme in animal hoarders than in object hoarders, given the extreme squalor and highly unsanitary conditions in which most animal hoarders live. Animal hoarders are generally not aware that their behavior poses a problem. Many hold delusional beliefs about special abilities to communicate with, understand, and care for animals.

Developmental Course Animal as well as object hoarding tends to be chronic. Animal hoarders generally start later in life (possibly for logistic rather than psychological differences as children are rarely in a position to hoard animals), hoarding becomes more severe over time, and high recidivism rates are typical.

4.4.5 Types of Animal Hoarders

Patronek notes that if there is one unifying characteristic of animal hoarding it is the heterogeneity of the syndrome (2006). Animal hoarders show considerable variation in their motivations, their underlying psychopathology, and the precipitating factors that have led to their hoarding behavior. Together with a group of mental health, social service, and law enforcement workers, all experienced with a variety of hoarding cases, Patronek proposed that hoarding cases clustered into three distinct categories: overwhelmed caregivers, rescuers, and exploiters (2006).

Overwhelmed Caregivers Overwhelmed hoarders usually start out with being able to maintain an adequate standard of care until situational factors (medical impairments, loss of income, loss of a spouse, family tragedy, etc.) overwhelm their capacity to adequately meet the animals' needs. Animals are acquired passively, often through a failure to neuter or spay. Sometimes the individual becomes known in the neighborhood as someone who will take in unwanted animals, and animals are brought to them. These hoarders tend to be less delusional, minimizing rather than denying the compromised condition of the animals. They are often socially withdrawn, and this isolation may be a factor in their reluctance to seek help. When they are confronted they are more amenable to intervention than are rescuer- or exploiter-type hoarders.

Rescuing or Mission-Driven Hoarders A strong sense of mission to rescue animals until the number of animals eventually overwhelms their ability to care for them characterizes this group. Their fierce commitment that no animal is euthanized overrides their awareness and empathy for the animals' suffering. Patronek (2006) suggests these hoarders have an extreme fear of death. Their procurement tends to be more active than passive. Often masquerading as legitimate animal shelters, they create a network of enablers to facilitate their acquisition of more animals. They avoid authorities, are secretive about their home situation, and impede access. Their mission to rescue animals leads eventually to a compulsion to acquire and control them.

Exploitative Hoarders Animal-hoarding cases typified by exploiters are the most serious and difficult to resolve. These hoarders, who show features of antisocial personality disorder, seem indifferent to the animals' suffering; rather, the animals serve their need for power and control. They show traits on the psychopathy spectrum—they are cunning, articulate, manipulative, superficially charming but harbor no empathy for people or animals, and feel no guilt or remorse about the harm they have caused. They engage in active procurement of animals for whom they have no emotional connection. They reject authority, possess an inflated sense of their own expertise, and are the least responsive to treatment. Frost et al. (2015) note that the lack of emotional attachment to their animals places exploiters outside the parameters of most animal hoarders such that they may not fit the criteria for HD. Fortunately, exploiters are thought to be the least common type of animal hoarder (Patronek 2006).

4.4.6   How Do We Explain Animal Hoarding Disorder?

Researchers generally agree that there is not one overarching theory to explain all hoarding cases, but rather that this disorder derives from multiple biological, social, and psychological factors. With extensive research about the possible etiology of animal hoarding based on clinical interviews with hoarders, interactions with hoarders through the law, family member interviews, and case-report analyses, HARC concludes that animal hoarding, like object hoarding, "is likely a final common pathway from a variety of traumatic experiences which result in dysfunctional attachment styles to people and lead to compulsive and addictive behavior" (FAQs for Hoarding of Animals Research Consortium: Who are hoarders and why do they hoard animals? http://vet.tufts.edu/hoarding/faqs-hoarding/).

4.4.6.1 Biological Abnormalities
There is evidence to suggest a biological mechanism at work within hoarding behavior. Hoarding has been found to be more common in patients with schizophrenia, with dementia, and those with structural defects in the frontal cortical and anterior cingulate cortex (ACC) regions of the brain. Saldarriaga-Cantillo and Nieto (2015) note that 30–50 % of patients with hoarding behaviors present with frontal lobe dysfunction, frontotemporal dementia, or vascular dementia, and case studies have reported the onset of hoarding behavior after an insult to the executive function regions of the brain (Tolin 2011). A study by Anderson et al. (2005) revealed that there may be specific brain regions involved. Sudden-onset severe hoarding behavior was found in patients who had damage to the medial frontal region of the brain, but not to patients who had brain lesions elsewhere. Tolin (2011) notes that there may also be a genetic vulnerability to hoarding. In families with OCD, chromosome 14 has been implicated in hoarding behavior.

4.4.6.2 Distinct from Obsessive-Compulsive Disorder
Although hoarding was formerly classified as a subcategory of OCD in the DSM-IV, emerging evidence precipitated a change in the DSM-5 to give HD its own classification distinct from OCD. Hoarding prevalence has been estimated to be twice that

of OCD, and fully 82 % of hoarders do not meet the diagnostic criteria for OCD (Frost et al. 2011). Patients with other anxiety disorders are more likely to exhibit hoarding symptoms than are OCD patients (Tolin et al. 2011).

Although accumulation may occur in OCD, the underlying motivation differs. OCD sufferers often accumulate possessions as a direct consequence of fears of contamination or avoiding the onerous cleaning, checking, or washing rituals necessitated by decluttering. Further, with OCD patients, the behavior is generally unwanted, sufferers derive no pleasure from this accumulation, and excessive acquisition is generally not evident (Mataix-Cols et al. 2010). Looking specifically at animal hoarding, Campos-Lima et al. (2015) found no relationship between OCD and animal hoarding in a sample of 420 patients attending a university OCD clinic.

4.4.6.3 Dissociation, Delusional Disorder, and Dementia

Dissociation has been used as an explanatory model for hoarding behavior because of the hoarder's lack of insight and seeming obliviousness to squalor and egregious animal suffering. With dissociation, an individual may separate different aspects of an experience and fail to integrate thoughts, feelings, and events, as a protection from being overwhelmed. The individual protects his or her self-concept by remaining unaware of the separated portion—be that memories, thoughts, or emotions related to the trauma (Brown and Katcher 2001; Brown 2011). In a study with 305 college undergrads, Brown found a positive correlation between levels of pet attachment and dissociation (Brown 2011). Participants with particularly high levels of pet attachment were three times more likely to exhibit clinical levels of dissociation than were those with average levels of pet attachment.

Delusional disorder, a subheading in the DSM-5 under "Schizophrenia Spectrum and other Psychotic Disorders," is characterized by the presence of one or more delusions that persist for at least 1 month. The criteria note that apart from the direct impact of the delusions, psychosocial functioning may not be as seriously impaired as in other psychotic disorders and behavior is not obviously bizarre or odd. Some researchers have suggested that hoarders' lack of insight, indifference to squalor and animal suffering, and belief in their supernatural abilities to communicate with their animals may be an aspect of a delusional disorder (Frost et al. 2011; Steketee et al. 2011).

Dementia may be accompanied by hoarding behavior, although it is has not been identified specifically in animal hoarding (HARC 2015; Saldarriaga-Cantillo and Nieto 2015).

Still other researchers have suggested that hoarders' lack of insight may be overstated. Steketee and Frost (2014) note that what is often interpreted as lack of insight may actually be defensiveness against a profound and prolonged history of interpersonal conflict with family, friends, and authorities. This defensiveness plays itself out in the therapist's office when clients may well rebel against any perceived attempt to constrain or control their freedom (Steketee and Frost 2014).

4.4.6.4 Addiction Model

Hoarders appear to share many characteristics with individuals with addiction issues: poor impulse control, denial of the problem, not taking responsibility for the consequences of their actions, neglect of personal affairs, and preoccupation with the addicted substance. Animal hoarders often feel driven to acquire more animals even when there is a modicum of understanding that this will lead to severe negative consequences—emotionally, socially, financially, and psychologically (Frost et al. 2015).

4.4.6.5 Attachment Disturbances and Trauma

Formulated to explain an individual's tendency to form enduring bonds with specific others, Bowlby's attachment theory (1982, 1988) holds that infants are biologically predisposed to maintain proximity to an attachment figure and to emit attachment behaviors that solicit caretaking (smiling, clinging, cooing, and crying). Similarly, caregivers are hardwired to respond in kind with warmth, love, and protection. Whether hoarders see their animals as attachment figures (their secure base, and safe haven in times of stress, as in an adult peer-to-peer relationship), or whether the animals serve primarily as an object of caretaking, (as in a parent-to-child relationship) is not clear. Potentially, animals fulfill both roles for hoarders who have disturbed or insecure attachment strategies.

As Attachment Figures Researchers have proposed that animal hoarders, unable to form a secure attachment to another individual, see their animals as attachment figures that provide unconditional love and comfort. Patronek and Nathanson (2009) suggest that insecure attachment relationships may lead to an over-compensation in a child's attachment to animals. Animals may have provided a safe haven in an otherwise chaotic and abusive world. This fragment of security becomes distorted into a belief as adults that more animals will provide even greater security. This belief becomes critical to the hoarder's sense of self-concept, control, and their reason for living (Patronek 2006). Related to this, Tolin found that object-hoarding patients often describe their emotional reaction toward discarding as one of grief rather than of fear (2011). Saldarriaga-Cantillo and Nieto (2015) note that with animals, unlike objects, a reciprocal relationship may be established where the animal is able to respond to this need with warmth and affection. This helps explain why, without intervention, recidivism (i.e., the percentage of hoarders who reacquire animals after they have been removed by authorities) approaches 100 % (Frost et al. 2015).

Hoarders are more likely to report a greater number of lifetime traumatic events than do OCD patients (Cromer et al. 2007) and community controls (Hartl et al. 2005). Trauma in childhood and/or adulthood includes sexual abuse, parental abandonment, interpersonal violence, relationship difficulties, home invasions, and death or unexpected loss of loved ones. In some cases, the trauma can be a precipitating trigger for the onset of hoarding behavior (Tolin 2011).

Nathanson (2009) proposes that animal hoarders who are continually acquiring homeless animals may be using the animals to numb a void left by major losses of attachment figures (either actually or emotionally) in childhood and adolescence.

Objects of Caretaking   Animals may help those with dysfunctional attachment relationships fulfill a compulsive caretaking role. Bowlby (1982) described "compulsive caretaking" as giving care obsessively to a vulnerable individual who is perceived by the caretaker to have suffered loss or difficulty, whether or not this care is wanted or warranted. Often, the care is welcome at first, but invariably becomes over-controlling and oppressive.

In a study comparing animal hoarders with non-hoarding owners of multiple animals, animal hoarders were more likely to see their animals as possessing human qualities and to see them as members of the family, often referring to the animals as their children or grandchildren (Steketee et al. 2011). Animal hoarders may receive powerful positive feedback from their imagined role as caretaker, protector, and provider and this reinforcement may drive the hoarding behavior (Flores 2004). Flores (2004) provides a convincing argument about how insecure or disorganized attachment to caregivers in childhood leaves a person vulnerable to addictive behaviors in adulthood in an effort to repair. Further, Young (2005) discusses how accumulation and control may be utilized to ameliorate psychological pain, but how ultimately these attempts only further diminish one's sense of self. Individuals with insecure, disorganized, or disordered attachment may still see themselves as providing a caregiving role, while in reality very little care is being given.

Mentalization has been described as a form of emotional knowledge that allows an individual to perceive and interpret the reality of others in terms of internal mental states such as needs, desires, feelings, and beliefs (Allen and Fonagy 2014). Securely attached individuals tend to have had caregivers with sophisticated mentalizing abilities who give feedback to their children about their child's and other's experiences, thus providing a model for children to reflect upon and understand their own and others' states of mind. Those with a history of disrupted attachment relationships, on the other hand, who have not received this modeling or feedback, may have an impaired ability to mentalize and do not recognize their own thoughts, feelings, or intentions, nor those of others (Allen and Fonagy 2014). Oblivious to others' mental states, they may volunteer unrestrained projection about the mental states of others. This mentalization deficit may be one mechanism that maintains hoarding behavior (Frost et al. 2015). The animal hoarder with impaired mentalization and insensible to the distress of their animals may accredit them with any mental state they wish ("The animals need me and love me," even when the animals are clearly suffering), or make up their own rules as to what constitutes distress (Patronek and Weis 2012).

4.4.6.6 Self-Psychology Model

Brown (2011) discusses the question of how animal hoarders typically claim to cherish the animals they are torturing through the lens of self-psychology. In self-psychology, the *self* (a personality structure that provides an individual with a sense of self-esteem, well-being, and cohesion) is maintained through interactions with people, animals, things, experiences, and ideas that are soothing and affirming—so called *self-objects*. According to Kohut (1971), it is the individual's perception of what they are receiving from the object that is critical rather than what the self-object may or may not be actually demonstrating. For the animal hoarder, the perceived feeling of being loved may still satisfy the psychological function of feeling validated even in the extreme situation where the animal has already died. Brown argues that this may in part explain how hoarded animals become a hoarder's essential reason for living, in spite of the fact that the animal's welfare is catastrophic.

Brown notes also that animal hoarders are likely to be stuck in *archaic* rather than *mature self-object relating*. Incapable of true empathy, they see the animal as an extension of themselves rather than as a being that has unique needs, desires, or perspectives. Hoarders' attempts to rescue these animals and provide for their safety may be an extension of their own feelings of insecurity and fear, leaving them unable to see the actual suffering that they are causing the animal (Brown 2011). Instead, they merge with the animal in order to confirm their sense of self-worth. Brown notes that animals lend themselves to being ideal *merger self-objects*. Since they cannot assert their own intentions, hoarders' projected emotions can easily be merged with that of the animal. Finally, through *disavowal*, animal hoarders are able to hold conflicting experiences side by side, are aware of these two parts of this double life, and keep their unacceptable home situation well hidden from the outside world. They retain a connection to reality in understanding that their behavior is unacceptable, while remaining bewildered by the motivating forces behind it and confirmed in the knowledge that the hoarding is vital to their existence.

4.4.6.7 Self-Neglect

Nathanson proposes that animal hoarding may well be one component of overall self-neglect (2009). Elderly people face a monumental challenge in maintaining a sense of value and personal control given the increasing threats to these aspects of self as they age. Self-neglect may reflect a last stronghold where the aging person can choose to maintain or disregard their personal care or maintenance of a clean and functional home (Nathanson 2009). While self-neglect may co-occur with mental or physical illness, Nathanson offers the disturbing notion that self-neglect may well emerge from the cumulative losses associated with normal aging. Children moving away, death of friends, loss of one's home, income, and status may all contribute to an elderly person's sense of obsolescence and redundancy. She suggests that in the case of the animal hoarder, the functional nature of the relationship between an isolated person and their animals to foster a sense of security and mutual nurturance eventually becomes dysfunctional. The animal becomes a readily accessible haven of safety and belonging that in a pathological sense can help the individual out of a traumatic situation such as grief or social abandonment (Saldarriaga-Cantillo and Nieto 2015). Self-neglecters typically report few or no attachment relationships and a history of negative social interactions with others where they felt abandoned, betrayed, or alienated.

Increasingly isolated, hoarders have no reality marker to confront their deteriorating living situation and alert them to the risks involved in their behavior (risk of losing their animals, their home, facing criminal charges, etc.). Nathanson suggests that the apparent "difficulty" that animal hoarders have in taking the perspective of another may be purposefully self-protective, allowing them to continue to hide from information that is confrontational and potentially discredits their sense of self and/ or dwindling control. This denial in turn allows animal hoarders to become rooted in a behavior that is extraordinarily resistant to change (Nathanson 2009).

4.4.7   Interventions

To date, there are no validated psychological interventions for animal hoarders specifically, but there exists an extensive and ongoing outcome research literature exploring effective treatments for object hoarders (e.g., Tolin 2011; Tolin et al. 2015), much of which can be extrapolated to animal hoarders. Recommendations from clinicians working with animal hoarders focus on recognizing the social isolation animal hoarders often experience, identifying and working on goals that matter to them, and addressing issues related to loss and attachment relationships. Interventions will necessarily vary according to the typology of the hoarder, with some types more amenable to treatment than others. Below are some potential issues relevant to most animal hoarders and guidelines for intervention (Nathanson 2009; Muroff et al. 2014):

4.4.7.1   Issues and Guidelines

1. Therapeutic alliance: Therapists need to be aware of how animal hoarders think about and explain their behavior and anticipate that the hoarder may have strongly held, but delusional beliefs. Nathanson (2009) argues that cultivating a relationship with the animal hoarder that recognizes their values, fears, and diminishing sense of self and control will facilitate the necessary alliance for rehabilitation to begin.
   (a) Hypervigilance and an exaggerated perception to threat make animal hoarders wary of authorities or anyone offering "help," which is perceived as a means to downsize or to intervene in their small kingdom of control. Patronek and Nathanson comment that overcoming this resistance with a distrusting individual, whose primary relationship has been with animals, poses a major challenge to establishing a therapeutic alliance (2009).
2. Interventions demand high investment and provide modest returns:
   (a) Most hoarders have poor insight, low motivation, high ambivalence, and treatment-resistant behaviors. Thus, interventions are likely to be long term. Once initiated, a treatment plan may be complicated by a hoarder's cognitive impairments, such as poor abstract reasoning, difficulty understanding cause and effect, poor problem-solving skills, and difficulty organizing, planning, and executing a task (Patronek and Nathanson 2009). Even with a cooperative patient, in an ideal situation, long-term support and ongoing monitoring of compliance will be necessary to bring about significant behavioral change.

    (b) Since hoarders are rarely self-referred, clinicians should expect motivational challenges such as poor compliance, missed appointments, and poor homework adherence. Because of this treatment resistance, harm reduction rather than symptom reduction may be a more appropriate treatment goal (Tolin 2011).

    (c) Simply removing animals is not an effective intervention as animal hoarders will typically accumulate more animals and soon find themselves in a similar situation to that of pre-intervention (Frost and Steketee 2014).

3. Interventions may need to vary according to the type of hoarder:

    (a) *Overwhelmed hoarders* may benefit from interventions to help them reduce the number of animals; there is the greatest likelihood for successful intervention from this group.

    (b) *Rescue hoarders* may need to be made aware of legal ramifications.

    (c) *Exploitative hoarders*, who have the least likelihood of rehabilitation, may need to be prosecuted.

4. Attachment disorder and/or attachment disturbances are likely:

Hoarders often have disturbed childhood attachment relationships. This is often exacerbated by an adult history of attachment figures (such as family members or friends) who have violated their trust by having the hoarder's animals removed (Patronek and Nathanson 2009). Clinicians will need to explore attachment-related issues such as loss, complicated grief, vulnerability, and social isolation, which may be significant in mitigating the animal-hoarding behavior (Patronek and Nathanson 2009).

5. Risk of suicide:

Because hoarders can experience profound grief reactions upon the removal of animals, clinicians will need to consider the potential suicide risk of hoarders. Veterinarians have noted that a client's bringing in multiple animals for euthanasia may be an incipient warning sign for suicide; they should be trained to recognize this behavior and make appropriate referrals to community mental health agencies.

6. Challenging delusional beliefs: Challenging hoarders' delusional beliefs is a necessary part of therapy. However, animal hoarders often show profound deficits in metacognition (the ability to reflect on one's own and other's thought processes), which poses limitations on the extent that the patient's own distorted beliefs can be confronted and redirected (Frost and Steketee 2014).

7. Comorbid disorders must be addressed: It is likely that animal hoarders are suffering from one or several other psychological disorders. Several conditions show elevated rates of comorbidity with HD: depression (50.7 %), social anxiety (23.5 %), OCD (18 %), attention-deficit disorder (28 %) (Frost et al. 2011), and perfectionism (Muroff et al. 2014). These disorders may well have a negative impact upon treatment delivery, patient adherence, and outcomes. Intervention into these other domains will be critical to the successful recovery of the animal hoarder.

8. Interventions will be multidisciplinary: Working with animal hoarding requires the integration of a range of different agencies including housing, environmental

health, social services, police, fire, mental health, and animal welfare. These may be disciplines that have not often worked together, and reciprocal education will be necessary.

9. A thorough neuropsychological evaluation may be advised as issues of competence, informed consent to treatment, and harm reduction need to be evaluated in the context of biological and neurological deficits (Tolin 2011).

4.4.7.2 Specific Intervention Strategies

Psychopharmacology Selective serotonin reuptake inhibitors (SSRIs) have been used with some success for obsessive-compulsive disorder, but results are mixed regarding their effectiveness for HD (Tolin 2011). Tolin, who has been a leader in outcome studies for HD treatments, including CBT and medication, believes that SSRIs should be considered, but that clinicians should have modest expectations about their effectiveness (2011).

Saxena et al. (2007), however, offer a more promising picture for the role of SSRIs in treating HD. In an outcome study looking at the effects of a 12-week trial of SSRIs, with no other medication or psychotherapy permitted during the trial, these researchers found that compulsive hoarders responded equally well to the SSRI paroxetine (Paxil) as nonhoarding OCD patients (Saxena et al. 2007). They demonstrated a 31 % decrease of hoarding behaviors, with significant and nearly identical improvements in OCD symptoms, depression, anxiety, and overall functioning. An ongoing study with the same research group found even more promising responses with the SSRI venlafaxine (Effexor XR). Preliminary data from 13 cases showed significant improvements in compulsive hoarding symptoms (a decrease of 37 %), as well as depressive, anxiety, and OCD symptoms. These authors suggest that venlafaxine may prove to be an effective treatment for HD; the target dose appears to be better tolerated by more patients, with fewer side effects than other SSRIs particularly for an older population (Saxena et al. 2007). To date, there have been no studies examining the efficacy of SSRIs for animal hoarding.

Cognitive Behavioral Therapy (CBT) Tolin (2011) suggests that CBT, specifically tailored for hoarders, needs to be a first line of defense. Traditional CBT used for OCD sufferers has had disappointing results, with OCD patients with a hoarding component demonstrating poorer outcomes than those with OCD alone. In a meta-analysis of 114 studies exploring the pre-to-posttreatment effect of CBT on HD overall severity, and specifically at the three core domains of acquiring, clutter, and difficulty discarding, Tolin et al. (2015) found a large effect of CBT on HD severity. The strongest effect was demonstrated with difficulty discarding, considered to be the core behavioral feature of HD. Moderate effects were also found for acquiring and clutter. Looking at these same domains (total HD severity, acquiring, clutter, and difficulty discarding), he also found that better outcomes were more likely in women, patients who were younger, those who were on psychiatric medication, who had a greater number of therapy sessions, and who had more home visits.

In a study of 46 patients randomly assigned to a CBT treatment group or a Waitlist (WL), Steketee et al. (2010) found that CBT patients improved significantly over WL patients in hoarding severity and mood at week 12. After 26 sessions, CBT participants showed significant reductions in hoarding symptoms: 41 % were clinically significantly improved, 71 % were considered improved based on therapists ratings, and 81 % considered themselves to have improved. The CBT was specifically designed to target hoarding symptoms and included motivational interviewing (e.g., homework adherence, attendance, etc.); skill training for organization, decision making, and problem solving; exposure to resisting acquisition and discarding; and challenging faulty cognitive beliefs about hoarding. A treatment plan was decided at the initial session but applied flexibly according to each patient's progress. Homework was decided at each session and patients were required to practice methods introduced in therapy at least three times per week. The last two sessions focused on relapse prevention and strategies to manage stressors without reverting to former maladaptive coping methods. Later in the therapy, after patients had learned specific skills, eight participants received one or two in-home sessions of 3–6 h where the patient worked hands on with the therapist sorting, organizing, and discarding. All decisions about what to discard were made according to the patients' rules.

Group Cognitive Behavior Therapy (GCBT) Muroff et al. (2009) demonstrated modest success using CBT in-group sessions (weekly for 16–20 weeks and two 90 min individual home visits) in 32 patients diagnosed with HD. Weekly group treatments focused on the following issues in approximately this progression:

1. Education about HD and the CBT model of therapy as way to understand hoarding symptoms
2. Introducing cognitive strategies to change beliefs about hoarding such as thinking errors and taking another's perspective
3. Emotion training and understanding attachment to possessions
4. Motivational enhancement strategies
5. Decision making and organization around clutter
6. Replacement of acquiring with more adaptive strategies using behavioral reinforcement; identification of roadblocks to progress
7. Exposure to sorting and discarding
8. Reducing acquisition
9. Involvement of family and/or coaches
10. Maintaining gains and preventing relapses; coping with improvement
11. Ending therapy

In a follow-up 20-week intervention outcome study, comparing GCBT to bibliotherapy—where patients read a self-help CBT treatment book during the same time period—Muroff et al. found significant reductions in hoarding and depressive symptoms evidenced in the GCBT group, whereas there was only minimal change in the bibliotherapy group. Benefits of GCBT were similar to individual CBT discussed in previous research (Muroff et al. 2012).

The authors note that group treatment may be of particular value to hoarding patients. It is cost-effective, offers patients greater access to clinicians trained in HD, reduces social isolation, and the social networking benefits of group therapy (offering mutual support, group cohesion, and social collaboration) improve motivation in a population where motivation has typically been a major roadblock to effective intervention. However, group therapy can sometimes undermine motivation, when individuals feel discouraged by not measuring up, or by focusing more effort and resources on others as a way of avoiding their own struggles, and that clinicians need to be cognizant of this possibility (Muroff et al. 2009).

Cognitive Remediation Training Cognitive remediation training (CRT) or cognitive enhancement training (CET) is a behavioral training intervention with the goal of improving cognitive processes such as attention, memory, executive function, social cognition, and metacognition. Research has provided promising results for CRT in patients with schizophrenia (e.g., Wykes et al. 2012), with effects lasting up to 6 months posttreatment (Kurtz et al. 2009), and these cognitive gains can be transferred to improvements in social and occupational functioning (Kurtz et al. 2009).

Highlights from Steketee and Frost's (2014), "Treatment for Hoarding Disorder: Therapist's Guide." In their comprehensive manual, Steketee and Frost (2014) propose a cognitive behavioral treatment plan specifically tailored to the hoarder's key issues of acquisition, clutter, and difficulty discarding. Steketee and Frost note that gaining control over compulsive acquisition is generally more easily attained than discarding items. Presumably, this would be even more salient for the animal hoarder where the "item" is a live animal that brings with it more complex issues of attachment and loss. The authors acknowledge that their manual has not been validated nor designed for animal hoarders; nevertheless, many of the suggested interventions address concerns that are common to both object and animal hoarders. In the absence of validated outcome research for animal hoarders, Steketee and Frost's manual provides a logical starting point:

Overview of sessions: Steketee and Frost suggest 26 sessions over 6-months – varying from 15 to more than 30 for severe cases. Sessions involve: assessment (2-3 sessions); case formulation (2 sessions); practice limiting the acquiring of objects (2-3 sessions); skills training (2-3 sessions) which includes problem-solving and organizational skills; sorting and discarding practice (15 sessions); and relapse prevention (final 2 sessions). Motivational interviewing is used throughout to address ambivalence about adherence and low insight.

Home visits: Key to their program are monthly home-visits of several hours. Steketee and Frost suggest that the first home visit occurs as the second session, if the client is amenable. This initial visit allows the clinician to determine the degree of clutter and squalor, whether the home poses an immediate safety threat, and potentially meet with family members. They recommend photographing all rooms to provide a baseline assessment and for reference throughout therapy. Photographs can help discouraged clients see visible progress from these initial images. Since clients will likely be embarrassed (many hoarding clients have not had visitors for years) and threatened (previous visits from family members or authorities may likely have resulted in the loss of their belongings), they suggest describing the goals of the home visit in a way that will allay their fears:

The home visit is very important for us to understand your thoughts and experiences about the things you own. So far I've asked you a lot of questions about the hoarding problem during this office visit. When we are at your home, I'll be asking how you feel and think about your things as you actually look at them and also what you typically do at home and how the clutter affects this. We can take pictures of your home to use during treatment to decide on next steps and to track your progress. The home visit helps me understand how you think and feel about your home and your things. Do you have any questions about the process or about anything else so far? (Steketee and Frost 2014, Chapter 3)

Steketee and Frost note that home visits tend to enhance motivation because of the progress that can be made in one session. Home visits may also be conducted by "coaches" – supportive and reliable friends or family members, or professional organizers whom the hoarder trusts. Clearly, animal hoarding poses a unique situation, as animals cannot simply be discarded. However, home visits can address the associated clutter and squalor evident in most animal hoarders' homes, and explore hoarders' relationship to their animals on site.

Client workbook: Steketee and Frost (2014) also provide a client workbook which they see as a critical aspect of therapy. Workbooks are used for recording homework, thoughts and beliefs, and treatment goals, and include organizing plans, cognitive techniques, and interventions used during treatment. Clinicians are encouraged to refer to the workbook often and to discuss with clients where the workbook will be kept, as items are easily lost in the hoarder's home.

Ongoing assessment through standardized measures: These authors also recommend using standardized measures which are included in their appendices to assess the type and severity of hoarding symptoms. Where available, measures include comparison scores of typical hoarders as well as control community samples, and suggest optimal cut-off scores for distinguishing clinically significant hoarding. Any of the measures can be completed by the client or the clinician. Significant discrepancies provide added information about the client's insight and delusional beliefs:

1. Hoarding Rating Scale (HRS: Tolin, Frost, & Steketee, 2010b, in Steketee and Frost 2014): This five-item scale, administered as a self-report or an interview, addresses key features of hoarding: Acquisition, Clutter, Difficulty Discarding, Distress, and Interference.
2. Saving Inventory-Revised (SI-R: Frost, Steketee, & Grisham, 2004, in Steketee and Frost 2014). This 23-item scale includes three subscales of Acquisition, Clutter, and Difficulty Discarding.
3. Clutter Image Rating (CIR: Frost, Steketee, Tolin, & Renaud, 2008, in Steketee and Frost 2014) is a 9-image pictorial measure varying from no clutter to severe clutter for a kitchen, living room, and bedroom. Clients select the picture that mostly closely resembles their own situation.
4. Saving Cognitions Inventory (SCI: Steketee, Frost & Kyrios, 2003, in Steketee and Frost 2014). This is a 24-item self-report assessing clients' attitudes and beliefs around discarding, including such issues as emotional attachment, responsibility, and need for control.
5. Activities of Daily Living (ADL-H: Frost, Hristova, Steketee, & Tolin, 2013 in Steketee and Frost 2014): This 15-item scale addresses to what degree the clutter impairs with the client's ability to complete ordinary activities of daily living such as cooking, bathing, and dressing.
6. Safety Questions: These questions help identify situations that compromise the safety of the hoarder's home such as fire hazards, blocked exits, and access by emergency personnel, and are graded on a scale of 0 = none to minimal to 5 = extreme.
7. Home Environment Index (Rasmussen et al., under review, in Steketee and Frost 2014). This 15-item scale provides a measure of the severity of squalor in the home.

Conceptual model: Steketee and Frost propose a conceptual model to describe the etiology and contributing factors of hoarding behavior. They suggest that:

1. Difficulties with acquisition, clutter, and discarding arise from personal vulnerabilities (perfectionism, dependency, negative mood, distorted core beliefs, and information processing problems such as perception, attention, memory, and decision-making).
2. These vulnerabilities contribute to hoarders' distorted beliefs about possessions (e.g., that they provide safety and comfort, or that they have inherent beauty and value), which in turn result in both positive and negative emotional responses that trigger hoarding behaviors.
3. These behaviors are positively reinforced through the pleasure gained by acquiring, and negatively reinforced through the avoidance of negative emotions such as grief, anxiety, or guilt (Steketee and Frost 2014).

Central to their therapy is the process of building this model with clients to identify their particular vulnerabilities, emotions, and hoarding behaviors. They suggest working with clients to develop two types of models: (1) a general conceptual model that incorporates all aspects of the hoarding problem that can be used for reference during the therapy, providing clients a way to understand their behavior and (2) a specific functional analysis that describes individual episodes of acquiring or difficulty discarding in real time to help clients understand their behavior in a specific instance. The authors provide sample case vignettes to illustrate how therapist and client might create these models together.

Motivational Interviewing: The hoarding patient's lack of insight about their problems and their low motivation to resolve them makes motivational interviewing strategies a key component of therapy (Tolin 2011). Tolin also notes that poor cooperation and adherence to homework is typical of hoarders and suggests that any move in this direction needs consistent positive reinforcement, whereas compliance failures need to be addressed and examined in therapy.

Steketee and Frost (2014) suggest that motivational strategies should be used whenever clients demonstrate ambivalence about the work and when that ambivalence is negatively impacting progress. This often occurs after the novelty of therapy has worn off and the client faces difficult decisions. They propose the motivational interviewing model outlined by Miller and Rollnick (2013) that assumes a person-centered intervention using compassion, partnership, and acceptance to strengthen the client's own motivation and capacity to change (Miller and Rollnick 2013, in Steketee and Frost 2014).

According to Miller and Rollnick, motivation to change is dependent upon two central themes: (1) the importance of change—the discrepancy between what life is like now and what the client would like it to be, and (2) a belief that change is possible—i.e., the confidence that the client will be able to effect this change. The therapist's job is to develop discrepancy—the importance of change—while drawing on the client's strengths to give them the confidence that they have the right and capacity to make informed choices. Developing discrepancy may be as simple as having the client visualize what it would be like to have a friend visit their home now, and a future visit when their home was free of clutter. Similarly, discrepancy can be developed by using the client's values and goals outlined at the beginning of therapy against their current reality—e.g., a grandparent who sees family as the highest priority, but cannot have her grandchildren to visit because her home is not safe (Steketee and Frost 2014). Steketee and Frost outline the basic assumptions of motivational interviewing that forms the foundation of the therapy:

1. *Motivation to change cannot be imposed by others*: Clients who enter treatment because they have been pressured to do so by family and friends are unlikely to respond favorably unless they first decide that treatment would benefit them personally.
2. *Ambivalence to change must be addressed*: Noncompliance and lack of common goals between therapist and client will undermine treatment; ambivalence must be addressed. Clients may express ambivalence through arriving late, canceling, and "forgetting" appointments, nonverbal signs of ambivalence, arguing, complaining, poor homework adherence, discounting progress, etc.
3. *Avoid direct persuasion*: The goal is for clients to explore and resolve their ambivalence rather than being convinced or persuaded by the therapist. Therapists need to be curious about ambivalence—drawing the client out to explore resistance—rather than moving into an authoritarian or persuasive role.
4. *Develop a trusting relationship*: Clients who have had their freedom of choice trampled by family, friends, and authorities are naturally mistrustful about the intentions of any intervention. Developing trust and a helpful working relationship takes time but is an essential component of motivational change.
5. *Therapy is a partnership*: Therapists elicit clients' *own* motivation to change, working with them to develop a commitment to change and an action plan to get there.

Mentalization-Based Treatment (MBT) MBT has been defined as a model of psychodynamic therapy grounded in attachment theory with the goal of enhancing the client's capacity to represent their thoughts, feelings, beliefs, and desires about themselves and significant others in the context of attachment relationships (Fonagy and Bateman 2008). Although initially conceived as a treatment for sufferers of borderline personality disorder (e.g., Bateman and Fonagy 2008; Fonagy and Bateman 2008), MBT has been more recently successfully applied to other clinical populations (e.g., Robinson et al. 2014) and has been proposed as an appropriate therapy for those with HD (Patronek and Weis 2012). In MBT, the focus of treatment centers on the mind of the patient. Patients learn about how they think and feel about themselves and others, how those thoughts and feelings govern their responses, and how these errors in understanding lead to actions that attempt to redeem stability and make sense of incomprehensible feelings (Bateman and Fonagy 2008).

Bateman and Fonagy outline the three-step process that underlies the structure and goals of MBT (2008):

1. *Assessment*: Assessing the patient's current capacity for mentalizing and personality function and inviting the patient to engage in treatment. Processes may include providing a diagnosis, education about MBT and the patient's psychological disorder, establishing a hierarchy of therapeutic goals, stabilizing interpersonal and behavioral problems, reviewing medications, and defining a crisis intervention pathway. The formulation can be modified as new understandings emerge in the sessions.
2. *Increasing mentalizing abilities*: The aim of all the active therapeutic work is to stimulate the patient's ever-evolving mentalizing ability. Central to the work is the exploration of events as they occur in therapy and guiding the client to understand the processes (e.g., the examination of affective states before the event) that have led to the loss of mentalization (see Bateman and Fonagay 2008, for a more detailed account).
3. *Preparation for terminating*: Here, the therapist focuses on the feeling of loss associated with the end of treatment, strategizes about how to maintain gains and minimize relapse, and develops a tailored follow-up program.

4.4.8 Conclusion

Research about HD has exploded in the work leading up to and since the publication of the DSM-5 where HD was finally awarded its own chapter, distinct from OCD. Unfortunately, the DSM committee fell short of giving animal hoarding its own unique classification. Undoubtedly, both assessment and treatment options will expand as animal hoarding is recognized as a unique subcategory of HD, complete with its own set of challenges and triumphs for clinicians and sufferers.

4.4.9 Animal Hoarding References

Allen JG, Fonagy P (2014) Mentalizing in psychotherapy. In: Hales R, Yudofsky S, Stuart C, Weis L (eds) American psychiatric publishing textbook of psychiatry, 6th edn. American Psychiatric, Arlington, pp 1095–1118

American Psychiatric Association (eds) (2013) A diagnostic and statistical manual of mental disorders, 5th edn. American Psychiatric Association Publishing, Washington, DC

Anderson SW, Damsio H, Damsio AR (2005). A neural basis for collecting behaviour in humans. Brain 128:201–212

Arluke A, Frost R, Carter L, Edward M, Nathanson J, Patronek GJ, Papazian M, Steketee G (2002) Health implications of animal hoarding. Health Soc Work 27(2): 125–137

Bateman A, Fonagy P (2008) Mentalization-based treatment for BPD. Soc Work Ment Health 6(1–2):187–201

Bowlby J (1982/1969) Attachment and loss, vol 1. Attachment, 2nd edn. Basic, New York

Bowlby J (1988) A secure base. Basic, New York

Brown SE (2011) Theoretical concepts from self psychology applied to animal hoarding. Soc Anim 19(2):175–193

Brown SE, Katcher AH (2001) Pet attachment and dissociation. Soc Anim 9(25):41

Campos Lima AL, Torres AR, Yücel M, Harrison BJ, Moll J, Ferreira GM, Fontenelle LF (2015) Hoarding pet animals in obsessive-compulsive disorder. Acta Neuropsychiatr 27(1):8–13

Cromer KR, Schmidt NB, Murphy DL (2007) Do traumatic events influence the clinical expression of compulsive hoarding? Behav Res Ther 45(11):2581–2592

Flores PJ (2004) Addiction as an attachment disorder. Jason Aronson, Lanham

Fonagy P, Bateman A (2008) The development of borderline personality disorder – a mentalizing model. J Pers Disord 22:4–21

Frost RO, Steketee G (eds) (2014) The Oxford handbook of hoarding and acquiring. Oxford University Press, New York

Frost RO, Steketee G, Williams L (2000) Hoarding: a community health problem. Health Soc Care Community 8(4):229–335

Frost RO, Patronek G, Rosenfield E (2011) Comparison of object and animal hoarding. Depress Anxiety 28(10): 885–891

Frost RO, Patronek G, Arluke A, Steketee G (2015) The hoarding of animals: an update. Psychiatric Times 32(4):1–5

Hartl T, Duffany SR, Allen GJ, Steketee G, Frost RO (2005) Relationships among compulsive hoarding, trauma, and attention deficit/hyperactivity disorder. Behav Res Ther, 43(2):269–276

Hoarding of Animals Research Consortium (2015) http://vet.tufts.edu/hoarding/. Retrieved 6 June 2015

Kohut H (1971) The analysis of the self: a systematic approach to the psychoanalytic treatment of narcissistic personality disorders. International University, New York

Kurtz MM, Seltzer JC, Fujimoto M, Shagan DS, Wexler BE (2009) Predictors of change in life skills of schizophrenia after cognitive remediation. Schizophr Res 107(2/3):267–274

Mataix-Cols D, Frost RO, Pertusa A, Clark LA, Saxena S, Leckman JF, Stein DJ, Matsunaga H, Wilhelm S (2010) Hoarding disorder: a new diagnosis for DSM-V? Depress Anxiety 27:556–572

Miller WR, Rollnick S (2013) Motivational interviewing: helping people change, 3rd edn. Guilford, New York

Muroff J, Steketee G, Rasmussen J, Gibson A, Bratiotis C, Sorrentino C (2009) Group cognitive and behavioral treatment for compulsive hoarding: a preliminary trial. Depress Anxiety 26:634–640

Muroff J, Steketee G, Bratiotis C, Ross A (2012) Group cognitive and behavioural therapy and bibliotherapy for hoarding: a pilot trial. Depress Anxiety 29:597–604

Muroff, J, Steketee G, Frost RO, Tolin DF (2014) Cognitive behavior therapy for hoarding disorder: follow-up findings and predictors of outcome. Depress Anxiety 31:964–971

Nathanson J (2009) Animal hoarding: slipping into the darkness of co-morbid animal and self-neglect. J Elder Abuse Negl 21(4):307–324

Patronek GJ (2006) Animal hoarding: its roots and recognition. Vet Med 101(8):520–531

Patronek G, Nathanson J (2009) A theoretical perspective to inform assessment and treatment strategies for animal hoarders. Clin Psychol Rev 29:274–281

Patronek GJ, Weiss KJ (2012) Animal hoarding: a neglected problem at the intersection of psychiatry, veterinary medicine, and law. Findings from the Henderson House Workgroup. Poster presented at: American Psychology-Law Conference. Poster 117–164. San Juan, Puerto Rico, 2012

Robinson P, Barrett B, Bateman A, Hakeem AZ, Hellier J, Lemonsky F, Rutterford C, Schmidt U, Fonagy P (2014) Study protocol for a randomized controlled trial of mentalization based therapy against specialist supportive clinical management in patients with both eating disorders and symptoms of borderline personality disorder. BMC Psychiatry 14:51

Saldarriaga-Cantillo A, Nieto C (2015) Noah Syndrome: a variant of diogenes syndrome accompanied by animal hoarding practices. J Elder Abuse Negl 27:270–275

Saxena S, Brody AL, Maidment KM, Baxter LR Jr (2007) Paroxetine treatment of compulsive hoarding. J Psychiatr Res 41(6):481–487

Steketee G, Frost RO (2014) Treatment for hoarding disorder: a therapist guide, 2nd edn. Oxford University Press, New York

Steketee G, Frost RO, Tolin DF, Rasmussen J, Brown TA (2010) Wait-listed control trial of cognitive behavior therapy for hoarding disorder. Depress Anxiety 27(5):476–484

Steketee G, Gibson A, Frost RO, Alabiso J, Arluke A, Patronek G (2011) Characteristics and antecedents of people who hoard animals: an exploratory comparative interview study. Rev Gen Psychol Am Psychol Assoc 15(2):114–124

Tolin DF (2011) Understanding and treating hoarding: a biopsychosocial perspective. J Clin Psychol Sess 67(5):517–526

Tolin DF, Fitch KE, Frost RO, Steketee G (2010) Family informants perceptions of insight in compulsive hoarding. Cogn Ther Res 34(1):69–81

Tolin DF, Meunier SA, Frost RO, Steketee G (2010) Course of compulsive hoarding and its relationship to life events. Depress Anxiety 27(9):829–838

Tolin DF, Frost RO, Steketee G, Muroff J (2015) Cognitive behavioral therapy for hoarding disorder: a meta-analysis. Depress Anxiety 32(3):158–166

Wykes T, Reeder C, Huddy V, Taylor R, Wood H, Ghirasim N, Kontis D, Landau S (2012) Developing models of how cognitive improvements change functioning: mediation, moderation and moderated mediation. Schizoph Res 138:88–93

Young ME (2005) Attachment disorder: a distortion of self and its effects on relationships. Psychol Educ 42:10–13

References

American Psychiatric Association (1987) Diagnostic and statistical manual of mental disorders III-R. American Psychiatric Association, Washington, DC

American Psychiatric Association (2013) Diagnostic and statistical manual of mental disorders V. American Psychiatric Association, Washington, DC

American Veterinary Medical Association (2012) U.S. pet ownership & demographics sourcebook. American Veterinary Medical Association, Schaumburg

Animal Welfare Institute (2015) Animals and family violence. Retrieved from https://awionline.org/content/animals-family-violence

Animals and Society Institute (Producer) (2001) The AniCare model of treatment for adults [DVD]. Animals and Society Institute (Producer), Ann Arbor

Arbour R, Signal T, Taylor N (2009) Teaching kindness: the promise of humane education. Soc Anim 17:136–148

Archer J (2000) Sex differences in physically aggressive acts between heterosexual partners: a meta-analytic review. Aggress Violent Behav 7:313–351

Arizona State University (2015) Children and animals together assessment and intervention program. Retrieved from http://psychweb.cisat.jmu.edu/graysojh/pdfs/Volume101-CATProg%20 Desc_updated%201-2014.pdf

Arkow P (2015a) Recognizing and responding to cases of suspected animal cruelty, abuse and neglect: What the veterinarian needs to know. Vet Med Res Rep 6:349–359

Arkow P (2015b) Animal-assisted therapy and activities: a study and research resource guide for the use of companion animals in animal-assisted interventions, 11th edn. P. Arkow, Stratford

Arkow P, Lockwood R (2013) Definitions of animal cruelty, abuse and neglect. In: Brewster MP, Reyes CL (eds). Animal Cruelty: A Multidisciplinary Approach to Understanding. Durham, NC: Carolina Academic Press, pp. 3–24

Arkow P, Munro H (2008) The veterinary profession's roles in recognizing and preventing family violence: the experiences of the human medicine field and the development of diagnostic indicators of non-accidental injury. In: Ascione FR (ed) International handbook of animal abuse and cruelty: theory, research, and application. Purdue University Press, West Lafayette, pp 31–58

Arkow P, Boyden P, Patterson-Kane E (2011) Practical guidance for the effective response by veterinarians to suspected animal cruelty, abuse and neglect. American Veterinary Medical Association, Schaumburg

Arluke A (1997) Interviewer guides used in cruelty research. Anthrozöos 10:180–182

Arluke A, Levin J, Luke C, Ascione F (1999) Relationship of animal abuse to violence and other forms of anitisocial behavior. Journal of Interpersonal Violence 14(9):963–975

Ascione FR (1992) Enhancing children's attitudes about the humane treatment of animals: generalization to human-directed empathy. Anthrozöos 5(3):176–191

© Springer International Publishing Switzerland 2016

K. Shapiro, A.J.Z. Henderson, *The Identification, Assessment, and Treatment of Adults Who Abuse Animals: The AniCare Approach*,

DOI 10.1007/978-3-319-27362-4

109

Ascione FR (1993) Children who are cruel to animals: a review of research and implications for developmental psychopathology. Anthrozoös 6:226–247

Ascione FR (1998) Battered women's reports of their partners' and their children's cruelty to animals. J Emot Abus 1:119–133

Ascione FR (2000) Safe havens for pets: guidelines for programs sheltering pets for women who are battered. Geraldine R. Dodge Foundation, Morristown

Ascione FR (2001) Animal abuse and youth violence. Juvenile justice bulletin. Office of Juvenile Justice and Delinquency Prevention (OJJDP), Rockville

Ascione FR, Shapiro K (2009) People and animals, kindness and cruelty: research directions and policy implications. J Soc Issues 65:565–589

Ascione FR, Thompson TM, Black T (1997) Childhood cruelty to animals: assessing cruelty dimensions and motivations. Anthrozös 10:170–177

Ascione FR, Weber CV, Thompson TM, Heath J, Maruyama MK, Hayashi K (2007) Battered pets and domestic violence: animal abuse reported by women experiencing intimate violence and by nonabused women. Violence Against Women 13:354–373

Association for Pet Obesity Prevention (2015) An estimated 54% of dogs and cats in the United States are overweight or obese. Retrieved from (http://www.petobesityprevention.org/)

Babcock SL, Neihsl A (2006) Requirements of mandatory reporting of animal cruelty. J Am Vet Med Assoc 229:685–689

Balcombe J (2006) Pleasurable kingdom: animals and the nature of feeling good. MacMillan, New York

Becker K, Stuewig J, Herrera V, McCloskey L (2004) A study of firesetting and animal cruelty in children: family influences and adolescent outcomes. J Am Acad Child Adolesc Psychiatry 43(7):905–912

Bickerstaff G (2003) An exploration of animal abuse and animal abusers. Unpublished dissertation, State University of New York, Albany

Boat B (1995) The relationship between violence to children and violence to animals. J Interpers Violence 10:229–235

Boat B (1999) Abuse of children and abuse of animals: using the links to inform child assessment and protection. In: Ascione FR, Arkow P (eds) Child abuse, domestic violence, and animal abuse: linking the circles of compassion for prevention and intervention. Purdue University Press, West Lafayette, pp 83–100

Boat B (2014) Connections among adverse childhood experiences, exposure to animal cruelty and toxic stress: what do professionals need to consider? Natl Cent Prosecution Child Abuse Update 24(4):1–3

Bryant B (1982) An index of empathy for children and adolescents. Child Dev 53:413–425

California, Health and Safety Code Act of 2008. § 25990–25994

Carlisle-Frank P, Flanagan T (2006) Silent victims: recognizing and stopping abuse of the family pet. Anthrozoös 19:374–375

Chur-Hansen A, McArthur M, Winefield H, Hanieh E, Hazel S (2014) Animal-assisted interventions in children's hospitals: a critical review of the literature. Anthrozoös 27:5–18

Clayton S, Fraser J, Saunders C (2009) Zoo experiences: conversations, connections, and concern for animals. Zoo Biol 28:377–397

Colorado Link Project (2015) Animal cruelty specific evaluation. Retrieved from http://colorado-linkproject.com/assessment-and-intervention/animal-cruelty-evaluation/

Courtois C, Ford J (2009) Treating complex traumatic stress disorders: an evidence-based guide. Cambridge University, Cambridge

Csillik A (2013) Understanding motivational interviewing effectiveness: contributions from Rogers' client-centered approach. Humanist Psychol 41(4):350–363

Currie CL (2006) Animal cruelty by children exposed to domestic violence. Child Abuse Negl Int J 30:425–435

Dadds MR, Fraser JA (2006) Fire interest, fire setting and psychopathology in Australian children: a normative study. Aust N Z J Psychiatry 40(6–7):581–586

Davis M (1983) Measuring individual differences in empathy: evidence for a multidimensional approach. J Pers Soc Psychol 44:113–126

Decastro R, Gaspar A, Vicente L (2010) The evolving empathy: hardwired bases of human and non-human primate empathy. Psicologia 24(2):131–152

Delta Society (2010) Standards of practice for animal-assisted activities and therapy. Delta Society, Bellevue

Di Pellegrino G, Fadiga L, Fogassi L, Gallese V, Rizzolatti G (1992) Understanding motor events: a neurophysiological study. Exp Brain Res 91:176–180

Donovan J, Adams C (eds) (1996) Beyond animal rights: a feminist caring ethic for the treatment of animals. Continuum, New York

Douglas K, Hart S, Kropp P (2001) Validity of the Personality Assessment Inventory for forensic assessments. Int J Offender Ther Comp Criminol 45:183–197

Downey G, Feldman S, Ayduk O (2000) Rejection sensitivity and male violence in romantic relationships. Pers Relat 7:45–61

Duncan A, Thomas JC, Miller C (2005) Significance of family risk factors in development of childhood animal cruelty in adolescent boys with conduct problems. J Fam Violence 20:235–239

Dutton DG, Nicholls TL, Spidel A (2005) Female perpetrators of intimate abuse. J Offender Rehabil 41:1–31

Eisenberg N, Miller P (1987) The relation of empathy to prosocial and related behaviors. Psychol Bull 101:91–119

Eisenberg N, Strayer J (1987) Critical issues in the study of empathy. In: Eisenberg N, Strayer J (eds) Empathy and its development. Cambridge University, Cambridge, pp 3–13

Erlanger AC, Tsytsarev SV (2012) The relationship between empathy and personality in undergraduate students' attitudes toward nonhuman animal. Soc Anim 20:21–39

Febres J, Shorey RC, Brasfield H, Zucosky HC, Ninnemann A, Elmquist J, Bucossi MM, Andersen SM, Schonbrun YC, Stuart GL (2012) Adulthood animal abuse among women court-referred to batterer intervention programs. J Interpers Violence 27:3115–3126

Febres J, Brasfield H, Shorey RC, Elmquist J, Ninnemann A, Schonbrun YC, Temple JR, Recupero PR, Stuart GR (2014) Adulthood animal abuse among men arrested for domestic violence. Violence Against Women 20(9):1059–1077

Flynn CP (1999) Exploring the link between corporal punishment and children's cruelty to animals. J Marriage Fam 61:971–981

Flynn CP (2011) Examining the links between animal abuse and human violence. Crime Law Soc Change 55:453–468

Forensic Psychiatry.ca (2015) Risk assessment: actuarial instruments and structured clinical guides. Retrieved at http://www.forensicpsychiatry.ca/risk/instruments.htm

Francione G (1995) Animals, property, and the law. Temple University, Philadelphia

George D, Phillips M, Doty L, Umhau J, Rawlings R (2006) A model linking biology, behavior and psychiatric diagnoses in perpetrators of domestic violence. Med Hypotheses 67(2):345–353

Gerbasi K (2004) Gender and nonhuman animal cruelty convictions: data from petabuse.com. Soc Anim 4:359–364

Gergen M, Gergen K (1984) The social construction of narrative accounts. In: Gergen K, Gergen M (eds) Historical social psychology. Erlbaum, Hillsdale

Goetz J, Keltner D, Simon-Thomasazarus E (2010) Compassion: an evolutionary analysis and empirical review. Psychol Bull 136:351–374

Gullone E, Robertson N (2008) The relationship between bullying and animal abuse behaviors in adolescents: the importance of witnessing animal abuse. J Appl Dev Psychol 29:371–379

Gullone E, Volant A, Johnson J (2003) A comparison of the co-occurrence of family violence and animal abuse across violent and non-violent families. Aust J Psychol 55:184–202

Gupta M (2008) Functional links between intimate partner violence and animal abuse: personality features and representations of aggression. Soc Anim 16:223–242

Harbolt T, Ward T (2001) Teaming incarcerated youth with shelter dogs for a second chance. Soc Anim 9:177–182

Henry BC (2004) The relationship between animal cruelty, delinquency, and attitudes toward the treatment of nonhuman animals. Soc Anim 12(3):185–207

Henry BC (2006) Empathy, home environment, and attitudes toward animals in relation to animal abuse. Anthrozoös 19(1):17–34

Hensley C, Tallichet S (2009) Childhood and adolescent animal cruelty methods and their possible link to adult violent crimes. J Interpers Violence 24:147–158

Hensley C, Tallichet S, Dutkiewicz E (2012) The predictive value of childhood animal cruelty methods on later adult violence: examining demographic and situational correlates. Int J Ther Comp Criminol 56:281–295

Herbert P, Young K (2002) Tarasoff at 25. J Am Acad Psychiatry Law 30:275–281

Herzog H (1991) Beneficial effects of pet ownership on some aspects of human health. J R Soc Med 84:717–720

Herzog H (2011) The impact of pets on human health and psychological well-being: fact, fiction, or hypothesis? Curr Dir Psychol Sci 20:236–239

Hines D, Brown J, Dunning E (2007) Characteristics of callers to domestic violence helpline for men. J Fam Violence 22:63–72

Jory B, Anderson D (1999) Intimate justice II: fostering mutuality, reciprocity, and accommodation in the treatment of abuse. J Marital Fam Ther 25:349–363

Jory B, Randour M (1998) The AniCare model of treatment for animal abuse. Psychologists for the Ethical Treatment of Animals, Washington Grove, MD

Jory B, Anderson D, Greer C (1997) Intimate justice: confronting issues of accountability, respect, and freedom in treatment for abuse and violence. J Marital Fam Ther 23:399–419

Kansas, Crimes against the Public Morals 2009 § 21–4310

Kellert SR, Felthous AR (1985) Childhood cruelty toward animals among criminals and noncriminals. Hum Relat 38:1113–1129

Lefkowitz C, Pharia I, Prout M, Debiak D, Bleiberg J (2005) Animal-assisted prolonged exposure: a treatment for survivors of sexual assault suffering posttraumatic stress disorder. Soc Anim 13:275–296

Levin J, Arluke A (2013) Young adults feel more empathy for battered dogs than for other adults. Paper presented at Annual Meeting of American Sociological Association, New York City

Lewchanin S, Zimmerman E (2000) Clinical assessment of juvenile animal abuse. Biddle Publishing Company & Audenreed, Brunswick

Lockwood R (1998) Factors in the assessment of dangerousness in perpetrators of animal abuse. Humane Society of the United States: Unpublished report

Lofflin J (2006) Animal abuse: what practitioners need to know. Vet Med 101(8):506–518

Loring M, Bolden-Hines T (2004) Pet abuse by batterers as a means of coercing battered women into committing illegal behavior. J Emot Abus 4:27–37

Luke C, Arluke A, Levin J (1997) Cruelty to animals and other crimes: a study by the MSPCA and Northeastern University. Massachusetts Society for the Prevention of Cruelty to Animals, Boston

Magdol L, Moffit TE, Caspi A, Newman DL, Fagan J, Siva PA (1997) Gender differences in partner violence in a birth cohort of 21 year olds: bridging the gap between clinical and epidemiological approaches. J Consult Clin Psychol 65:68–78

Marino L (2012) Construct validity of animal assisted therapy and activities: how important is the animal in AAT? Anthrozoös 25(Supplement 1):139–151

McGoldrick M, Gerson R (1985) Genograms in family assessment. Norton, New York

McPhedran S (2009) Animal abuse, family violence, and child wellbeing: a review. Journal of Family Violence 24:41–52

Merz-Perez L, Heide KM, Silverman IJ (2001) Childhood cruelty to animals and subsequent violence against humans. Int J Offender Ther Comp Criminol 45:556–573

Midgley M (1983) Animals and why they matter: a journey around the species barrier. University of Georgia, Atlanta

Miller A (2014) Psychologists are leaders in the growing field of threat assessment. Monit Psychol 45:37–38

Miller W, Rollnick S (2002) Motivational interviewing: helping people change. Guilford, New York

Miller L, Zawistowski S (1997) A call for veterinary forensics: the preparation and interpretation of physical evidence for cruelty investigation and prosecution. In: American Humane Association (ed) A manual to aid veterinarians in preventing, recognizing, and verifying animal abuse, American Humane Association. American Humane Association, Englewood, pp 63–67

Moffitt T, Robins R, Caspi A (2001) A couples analysis of partner abuse with implications for abuse prevention. Criminol Public Policy 1:5–36

Mounoud P (1996) Perspective taking and belief attribution: from Piaget's theory to children's theory of mind. Swiss J Psychol 55:93–103

Munro HMC (1996) Battered pets. Ir Vet J 49:712–713

National Child Traumatic Stress Network (2015) Symptoms and behaviors associated with exposure to trauma. Retrieved from http://www.nctsn.org/trauma-types/early-childhood-trauma/Symptoms-and-Behaviors-Associated-with-Exposure-to-Trauma

National District Attorney Association (2015) Counseling laws for convicted animal abusers. Retrieved from http://www.ndaa.org/pdf/Counseling%20Laws%20for%20Convicted%20Animal%20Abusers%20-%20February%202013.pdf

National Link Coalition (2012) Toolkit for starting a link coalition in your community. National Link Coalition, Stratford

National Link Coalition (2015a) National link coalition. Retrieved from http://nationallinkcoalition.org/

National Link Coalition (2015b) Cross-reporting by type. National Link Coalition, Stratford

Nezu A, Nezu C, D'Zurilla T (2013) Problem-solving therapy: a treatment manual. Springer, New York

Nussbaum M (2011) Creating capabilities: the human development approach. Belknap, Cambridge, MA

Patronek G (1997) Issues for veterinarians. Soc Anim 5:267–280

Patronek GJ, Sacks JJ, Delise KM, Cleary DV, Marder AR (2013) Co-occurrence of potentially preventable factors in 256 dog bite-related fatalities in the United States (2000–2009). J Am Vet Med Assoc 243(12):1726–1736

Phillips H, Lockwood R (2013) Investigating & prosecuting animal abuse: a guidebook on safer communities, safer families & being an effective voice for animal victims. National District Attorneys Association, Alexandria

Piaget J (1926) The child's conception of the world. Translated by Totowa: Rowman and Allanheld, 1960. Originally published as La représentation du monde chez l'enfant. Paris: Presses Universitaires de France

Rajewski G (2015) CSI: animal abuse. Retrieved from http://now.tufts.edu/articles/csi-animal-abuse

Red Rover (2015) Red rover readers. Retrieved from http://redrover.org/program/redrover-readers

Regan T (1983) The case for animal rights. University of California, Berkeley

Rigdon JD, Tapia F (1977) Children who are cruel to animals: a follow-up study. J Oper Psychiatry 8:27–36

Rizzolatti G, Gallese V, Fadiga L, Fogassi L (1996) Action recognition in the premotor cortex. Brain 119:593–609

Rizzolatti G, Fogassi L, Gallese V (2006) Mirrors of the mind. Sci Am 295:54–61

Rockett B, Carr S (2014) Animals and attachment theory. Soc Anim 22:415–433

Rosenbaum A, Maiuro R (1989) Eclectic approaches in working with men who batter. In: Caesar PL, Hamberger LK (eds) Treating men who batter: theory, practice, and programs. Springer, New York, pp 165–195

Rowland M (1998) Animal rights: a philosophy defence. St. Martin's, New York

Ryder R (1975) Victims of science: the use of animals in research. Davis-Poytner, London

Serpell J (1986) In the company of animals: a study of human-animal relationships. Basil Blackwell, Oxford

Shapiro K (1990) Learning and unlearning empathy. Phenomenol Pedagog 8:43–49

Shapiro K (2008) Human-animal studies: growing the field, applying the field. Animals and Society Institute, Ann Arbor

Shapiro K, Randour M, Krinsk S, Wolf J (2014) The assessment and treatment of children who abuse animals: the AniCare child approach. Springer, New York

Shiota M, Keltner D, John O (2006) Positive emotion dispositions differentially associated with big five personality and attachment style. J Posit Psychol 1:61–71

Simmons CA, Lehmann P (2007) Exploring the link between pet abuse and controlling behaviors in violent relationships. J Interpers Violence 22:1211–1222

Singer P (1975) Animal liberation: a new ethic for our treatment of animals. Avon, New York

Sonkin D, Liebert D (2003) The assessment of court-mandated perpetrators of domestic violence. J Trauma Aggress Maltreat Trauma 6(2):3–36

Stets JE, Straus MA (1989) The marriage license as a hitting license: a comparison of assaults in dating, cohabiting, and married couples. J Fam Violence 4(2):161–180

Straus MA, Gelles RJ (1988) National survey on abuse of the elderly in Canada: preliminary findings. In: Hotaling GT, Finkelhor D, Kirkpatrick JT, Straus MA (eds) Family abuse and its consequences: new directions in research. Sage, Beverly Hills, pp 14–36

Stuart G, Meehan J, Moore T, Morean M, Hellmuth J, Follansbee K (2006) Examining a conceptual framework of intimate partner violence in men and women arrested for domestic violence. J Stud Alcohol 67(1):102–112

Tapia F (1971) Children who are cruel to animals. Child Psychiatry Hum Dev 2:70–77

Taylor N, Signal T (2006a) Community demographics and the tendency to report animal abuse. J Appl Anim Welf Sci 3:201–211

Taylor N, Signal T (2006b) Attitudes to animals in the animal protection movement compared to a normative community sample. Soc Anim 18:18–27

Thompson K, Gallone E (2006) An investigation into the association between the witnessing of animal abuse and adolescents' behavior toward animals. Soc Anim 14:221–244

University of Tennessee, Knoxville (2015) Veterinary social work. Retrieved from http://www.vetsocialwork.utk.edu/about.php

Upadhya V (2014) The abuse of animals as a method of domestic violence: the need for criminalization. Emory Law J 63:1163–1209

Vaughn MG, Fu Q, DeLisi M, Beaver KM, Perron BE, Terrell K, Howard MO (2009) Correlates of cruelty to animals in the United States: results from the national epidemiologic survey on alcohol and related conditions. J Psychiatr Res 43:1213–1218

Vaughn M, Salas-Wright C, DeLisi M, Larson M (2015) Deliberate self-harm and the nexus of violence, victimization, and mental health problems in the United States. Psychiatry Res 225:588–595

Vermeulen H, Odendaal J (1993) Proposed typology of companion animal abuse. Anthrozoös 6:248–257

Volant AM, Johnson JA, Gullone E (2008) The relationship between domestic violence and animal abuse: an Australian study. J Interpers Violence 23:1277–1295

Walters GD (2013) Testing the specificity postulate of the violence graduation hypothesis: meta-analyses of the animal cruelty offending relationship. Aggress Violent Behav 18:797–802

Weil Z (2004) The power and promise of humane education. New Society, Gabriola Island

White M (2007) Maps of narrative practice. Norton Professional Books, New York

White M, Epston D (1990) Narrative means to therapeutic ends. WW Norton, New York

Wright J, Hensley C (2003) From animal cruelty to serial murder: applying the graduation hypothesis. Int J Offender Ther Comp Criminol 47:71–88

Yorke J, Adams C, Coady N (2008) Therapeutic value of equine–human bonding in recovery from trauma. Anthrozoös 21:17–30

Zilcha-Mano S (2013) Animal-assisted psychotherapy from an attachment perspective. In: Parish-Plass N (ed) Animal-assisted psychotherapy: theory, issues, and practice. Purdue University, West Lafayette, pp 111–145